The Great Cancer Diet Cookbook: Healing Recipes and Meal Plans for Cancer Patients

Dr. Willis Cotton

Copyright

Foreword

Cancer is a journey no one anticipates, yet it is one that millions face each year. Amid the whirlwind of treatments, doctor visits, and emotional highs and lows, one aspect often remains a cornerstone of strength and healing: nutrition. The food we consume plays a critical role in supporting our bodies, boosting our immune systems, and enhancing our overall well-being.

This book, *The Great Cancer Diet Cookbook: Healing Recipes and Meal Plans for Cancer Patients,* is born out of a commitment to empower and support those on this challenging path. As a nutritionist and chef dedicated to the well-being of cancer patients, I have seen firsthand how the right foods can make a significant difference. This cookbook is a culmination of years of research, culinary expertise, and the heartfelt stories of those who have bravely faced cancer.

Inside, you will find recipes that are not only nourishing and delicious but also tailored to meet the unique needs of cancer patients. From combating treatment side effects like nausea and fatigue to fortifying the body with essential nutrients, each recipe is crafted with care and intention.

Moreover, this book offers more than just recipes. It provides meal plans designed to simplify the process of eating well during a time when energy and appetite may be compromised. Practical tips, dietary advice, and inspirational stories are woven throughout, making this cookbook a comprehensive guide for anyone looking to support their health through food.

Whether you are a cancer patient, a caregiver, or a loved one seeking ways to provide comfort and care, this book is for you. It is a testament to the resilience of the human spirit and the profound impact that good nutrition can have on the journey to healing.

May these pages offer you strength, hope, and the knowledge that you are not alone. Together, we can nourish our bodies and spirits, one meal at a time.

With heartfelt gratitude,

Dr. Michael Harper

Acknowledgments

Creating "The Great Cancer Diet Cookbook: Healing Recipes and Meal Plans for Cancer Patients" has been a deeply personal and fulfilling journey, and I am grateful to the many people who made this book possible.

First and foremost, I want to extend my heartfelt gratitude to the cancer patients and survivors who shared their experiences and insights. Your courage and resilience are the foundation of this cookbook.

A special thank you to the medical professionals, dietitians, and nutritionists who provided invaluable guidance and expertise. Your dedication to improving the lives of cancer patients is truly inspiring.

I am deeply appreciative of my family and friends for their unwavering support, encouragement, and patience throughout this process. Your love and belief in me were my greatest sources of strength.

To my editor, thank you for your meticulous attention to detail and thoughtful suggestions. Your expertise has significantly enhanced the quality of this book.

A sincere thank you to my recipe testers, whose feedback and enthusiasm ensured that each dish is both delicious and healing.

Lastly, to my readers, thank you for trusting me to be a part of your healing journey. It is my hope that this cookbook provides you with nourishment, comfort, and hope.

With gratitude,
Dr. Emilia Green

Table of Contents

8. Dinner
  - Balanced Main Courses
    - Baked Salmon with Asparagus
    - Quinoa-Stuffed Bell Peppers
  - Plant-Based Proteins
    - Chickpea and Spinach Curry
    - Black Bean and Sweet Potato Enchiladas
  - Healthy Side Dishes
    - Roasted Brussels Sprouts
    - Steamed Broccoli with Lemon

9. Snacks and Appetizers
  - Nutrient-Dense Snacks
    - Almond and Date Energy Balls
    - Veggie Chips
  - Healthy Dips and Spreads
    - Classic Hummus
    - Avocado and White Bean Dip
  - Simple Appetizers
    - Stuffed Mushrooms
    - Caprese Skewers

10. Desserts
  - Guilt-Free Treats
    - Dark Chocolate Avocado Mousse

Introduction

Cancer is a formidable adversary, impacting millions worldwide each year. While medical treatments are crucial, diet and nutrition play a pivotal role in cancer prevention, treatment, and recovery. "The Great Cancer Diet Cookbook: Healing Recipes and Meal Plans for Cancer Patients" is designed to be a comprehensive guide, offering scientifically-backed nutritional advice and delicious recipes to support cancer patients on their journey to health. This book aims to empower individuals with the knowledge and tools to make informed dietary choices, thereby enhancing their overall well-being.

Welcome to The Great Cancer Diet Cookbook

Welcome to "The Great Cancer Diet Cookbook," a resource dedicated to those seeking to harness the power of nutrition in their battle against cancer. This cookbook is not just about recipes; it's about a holistic approach to eating that supports the body's natural defenses, aids in recovery, and promotes long-term health. We understand that every cancer journey is unique, and so are the dietary needs and preferences of each individual. Our goal is to provide a versatile and accessible collection of recipes and meal plans that can be tailored to fit various needs.

Author's Journey and Motivation

The creation of this cookbook is deeply personal. As the author, my journey with cancer began when a close family member was diagnosed. Watching their struggle and witnessing the impact of diet on their well-being inspired me to delve into the science of nutrition and cancer. Through extensive research and collaboration with nutritionists, oncologists, and cancer survivors, I discovered the profound influence that specific foods can have on health outcomes. This book is a culmination of that journey—a blend of personal experience, scientific evidence, and culinary creativity aimed at providing practical support to others facing similar challenges.

My motivation is simple: to offer a beacon of hope and a practical guide for those navigating the tumultuous waters of cancer. I want to help others understand that they are not powerless and that the food they eat can be a powerful ally in their fight against cancer.

Purpose and Goals of This Book

The primary purpose of "The Great Cancer Diet Cookbook" is to serve as a reliable companion for cancer patients, their families, and caregivers. Here are the key goals of this book:

1. Provide Evidence-Based Nutrition Advice: Each recipe and meal plan is rooted in scientific research, focusing on ingredients known for their cancer-fighting properties.

2. Offer Practical Meal Solutions: We aim to simplify meal preparation with easy-to-follow recipes and tips for efficient cooking, ensuring that nutritious meals are accessible even during the most challenging times.

3. Address Specific Nutritional Needs: This book covers various aspects of cancer nutrition, including managing treatment side effects, boosting immunity, and maintaining overall health.

4. Empower Through Knowledge: By educating readers on the role of nutrition in cancer care, we hope to empower them to make informed dietary choices that support their health and recovery.

5. Create a Sense of Community: Through shared stories and testimonials, we aim to build a community of support and encouragement for all those affected by cancer.

How to Use This Cookbook

"The Great Cancer Diet Cookbook" is designed to be user-friendly and adaptable. Here's how you can make the most of it:

1. Start with the Basics: Begin by familiarizing yourself with the introduction and nutritional information sections. Understanding the foundation of cancer nutrition will help you make better dietary choices.

2. Explore the Recipes: The cookbook is divided into sections based on meal types—breakfast, lunch, dinner, snacks, desserts, and drinks. Each section offers a variety of recipes that cater to different tastes and dietary requirements.

3. Utilize Meal Plans: Use the sample meal plans provided as a guide. These plans are customizable and can be adjusted to meet individual preferences and nutritional needs.

4. Address Specific Needs: If you are dealing with particular side effects from treatment, refer to the special diets section. Here you will find recipes tailored to manage symptoms like nausea, mouth sores, and appetite loss.

5. Take Notes and Adapt: Don't hesitate to tweak recipes to better suit your taste or dietary needs. The cookbook is meant to be flexible and adaptable.

6. Join the Community: Engage with the stories and testimonials from other cancer survivors. Their experiences can provide motivation and a sense of solidarity.

Understanding Cancer and Nutrition

The relationship between cancer and nutrition is complex and multifaceted. Proper nutrition can support the body's natural defenses, enhance the effectiveness of treatments, and improve overall quality of life. Here are some key points to understand:

1. Cancer-Fighting Foods: Certain foods are rich in antioxidants, vitamins, and minerals that can help protect cells from damage, reduce inflammation, and inhibit the growth of cancer cells. Examples include leafy greens, berries, nuts, seeds, and fatty fish.

2. Nutrient-Dense Diet: A diet high in nutrient-dense foods provides the body with essential nutrients needed for healing and repair. This includes a balance of macronutrients (proteins, fats, and carbohydrates) and micronutrients (vitamins and minerals).

3. Managing Side Effects: Cancer treatments such as chemotherapy and radiation can cause side effects that impact nutrition, including nausea, appetite loss, and mouth sores. Tailored dietary strategies can help manage these symptoms and maintain nutritional intake.

4. Boosting Immunity: The immune system plays a crucial role in fighting cancer. Nutrients such as vitamin C, vitamin E, and zinc support immune function, while probiotics and prebiotics promote a healthy gut microbiome.

5. Maintaining Healthy Weight: Maintaining a healthy weight is important for overall health and recovery. This includes strategies for managing weight loss due to treatment side effects and avoiding excessive weight gain.

6. Hydration: Staying hydrated is vital, especially during treatment. Adequate fluid intake helps maintain bodily functions, supports detoxification, and can alleviate some treatment side effects.

7. Holistic Approach: Nutrition is just one aspect of a holistic approach to cancer care. Regular physical activity, stress management, and adequate sleep are also important components of overall health and well-being.

The Role of Diet in Cancer Care

Cancer is a multifaceted disease that affects millions of people worldwide. While medical treatments like chemotherapy, radiation, and surgery are crucial in battling cancer, nutrition plays an equally important role in prevention, treatment, and recovery. A well-planned diet can support the body's immune system, improve overall well-being, and potentially enhance the effectiveness of cancer treatments. "The Great Cancer Diet Cookbook: Healing Recipes and Meal Plans for Cancer Patients" provides an in-depth exploration of how diet impacts cancer care and offers practical guidance for making nutritious, cancer-fighting food choices.

How Nutrition Affects Cancer Prevention and Recovery

Nutrition is a critical factor in both cancer prevention and recovery. Numerous studies have shown that a healthy diet can reduce the risk of developing certain types of cancer and support the body during and after treatment. Here are several ways nutrition impacts cancer care:

1. **Immune System Support:** A diet rich in vitamins, minerals, and antioxidants helps strengthen the immune system, which is essential for preventing infections and aiding the body in fighting cancer cells. Nutrients such as vitamin C, vitamin E, and zinc are particularly important for immune function.

2.   Inflammation   Reduction: Chronic inflammation is a known risk factor for cancer. Anti-inflammatory foods like leafy greens, berries, and fatty fish contain compounds that help reduce inflammation and lower the risk of cancer.

3. Cellular Repair and Growth: Nutrients like protein, vitamins, and minerals are crucial for the repair and growth of healthy cells, especially after treatments like chemotherapy and radiation that can damage normal cells.

4. Managing Side Effects: Proper nutrition can help manage the side effects of cancer treatments. For example, foods that are easy to digest and high in nutrients can help mitigate nausea, appetite loss, and other gastrointestinal issues common during treatment.

5. Energy and Strength Maintenance: Cancer and its treatments can lead to fatigue and weakness. A diet that includes a balanced mix of proteins, carbohydrates, and fats provides the necessary energy to maintain strength and support recovery.

6. Weight Management: Maintaining a healthy weight is crucial for overall health and can improve treatment outcomes. A balanced diet helps prevent weight loss caused by treatment side effects or weight gain from inactivity and certain medications.

7. Mental Well-being: Nutrition also affects mental health, which is vital for overall well-being. Foods rich in omega-3 fatty acids, such as fish, and those high in antioxidants, like fruits and vegetables, can improve mood and cognitive function.

Overview of Cancer-Fighting Foods

Certain foods are known for their cancer-fighting properties due to their high content of antioxidants, phytochemicals, vitamins, and minerals. Including these foods in your diet can help reduce cancer risk and support recovery. Here's an overview of some of the most potent cancer-fighting foods:

1. Leafy Greens: Spinach, kale, and Swiss chard are rich in vitamins A, C, and K, as well as antioxidants that protect cells from damage. They also contain fiber, which aids in digestion and helps eliminate toxins from the body.

2. **Berries:** Blueberries, strawberries, and raspberries are packed with antioxidants, such as vitamin C and flavonoids, which help neutralize free radicals and reduce inflammation.

3. **Cruciferous Vegetables:** Broccoli, cauliflower, Brussels sprouts, and cabbage contain glucosinolates, which are compounds that have been shown to inhibit the growth of cancer cells and help in detoxifying harmful substances.

4. **Fatty Fish:** Salmon, mackerel, and sardines are excellent sources of omega-3 fatty acids, which have anti-inflammatory properties and can inhibit the growth of cancer cells.

5. Nuts and Seeds: Almonds, walnuts, chia seeds, and flaxseeds are rich in healthy fats, fiber, and antioxidants. They help reduce inflammation and support heart health.

6. Whole Grains: Brown rice, quinoa, barley, and oats provide fiber, vitamins, and minerals that support overall health and aid in maintaining a healthy weight.

7. Garlic and Onions: These allium vegetables contain sulfur compounds that boost the immune system and may reduce the risk of certain cancers, such as stomach and colorectal cancer.

8. Green Tea: Rich in polyphenols, particularly epigallocatechin gallate (EGCG), green tea has powerful antioxidant and anti-cancer properties.

9. Turmeric: This spice contains curcumin, which has strong anti-inflammatory and antioxidant effects. It has been shown to inhibit the growth of various cancer cells in studies.

10. Legumes: Beans, lentils, and peas are high in fiber, protein, and folate. They help regulate blood sugar levels and support digestive health, which is important for cancer prevention and recovery.

Foods to Avoid During Cancer Treatment

While certain foods can support cancer treatment and recovery, others can potentially hinder progress and exacerbate symptoms. It is crucial to be mindful of what to avoid to optimize health and well-being during cancer treatment:

1. **Processed Meats**: Hot dogs, sausages, and deli meats contain preservatives and nitrates that can increase the risk of certain cancers, particularly colorectal cancer. These meats are also often high in sodium, which can lead to dehydration and other health issues.

2. **Sugary Foods and Beverages**: Excessive sugar intake can lead to weight gain and inflammation. Sugary drinks and snacks

provide empty calories and can cause spikes in blood sugar levels, which may negatively impact energy and mood.

3. **Fried and Greasy Foods**: These foods are difficult to digest and can cause nausea, indigestion, and other gastrointestinal problems. They are also high in unhealthy fats, which can increase inflammation.

4. **Alcohol**: Alcohol can weaken the immune system and interfere with the effectiveness of cancer treatments. It also increases the risk of developing certain types of cancer, such as liver, breast, and esophageal cancer.

5. **Red Meat**: While lean red meat in moderation can be part of a healthy diet, excessive consumption has been linked to an increased risk of colorectal and other cancers. It is better to focus on plant-based proteins and fatty fish.

6. **Refined Carbohydrates**: White bread, white rice, and pastries are low in nutrients and high in refined sugars, which can contribute to

weight gain and inflammation. Whole grains are a healthier alternative.

7. **High-Sodium Foods**: Canned soups, processed snacks, and fast foods are often high in sodium, which can lead to dehydration and high blood pressure. Reducing sodium intake is essential for maintaining fluid balance and overall health.

8. **Artificial Additives and Preservatives**: Many processed foods contain artificial colors, flavors, and preservatives that can be harmful to health. These additives can cause allergic reactions, digestive issues, and potentially contribute to cancer risk.

9. **Dairy Products**: For some people, dairy can cause inflammation and digestive problems. If you notice discomfort after consuming dairy, consider plant-based alternatives like almond or soy milk.

10. **Raw or Undercooked Foods**: Cancer treatments can weaken the immune system, making it easier to contract foodborne

illnesses. It is important to avoid raw or undercooked meats, eggs, and seafood to reduce the risk of infection.

Importance of a Holistic Approach

A holistic approach to cancer care encompasses more than just dietary changes. It involves considering the whole person—mind, body, and spirit—and integrating various aspects of health to support overall well-being. Here are key elements of a holistic approach to cancer care:

1. **Physical Activity**: Regular exercise can help improve mood, reduce fatigue, and enhance overall physical health. Activities like walking, yoga, and swimming can be tailored to individual fitness levels and treatment schedules.

2. **Stress Management**: Chronic stress can weaken the immune system and negatively impact health. Techniques such as meditation, deep breathing exercises, and mindfulness

can help manage stress and promote relaxation.

3. **Adequate Sleep**: Quality sleep is essential for healing and recovery. Establishing a regular sleep routine and creating a restful environment can improve sleep quality and overall health.

4. **Emotional Support:** Emotional well-being is a critical component of holistic care. Support groups, counseling, and therapy can provide a safe space to express feelings and receive support from others who understand the cancer journey.

5. **Complementary Therapies**: Integrating complementary therapies like acupuncture, massage, and aromatherapy can help manage symptoms and improve quality of life. Always consult with healthcare providers before starting any new therapy.

6. **Spiritual Wellness**: For many, spirituality can be a source of strength and comfort during challenging times. Engaging in

spiritual practices, whether through religion, nature, or personal reflection, can provide a sense of peace and purpose.

7. **Hydration**: Staying hydrated is vital for overall health. Drinking plenty of water helps flush toxins from the body, supports digestion, and maintains energy levels. Herbal teas and infused waters can also be beneficial.

8. **Social Connections:** Maintaining strong social connections and engaging in social activities can improve mental health and provide emotional support. Spending time with family and friends, participating in community events, and joining support groups can foster a sense of belonging and reduce feelings of isolation.

9. **Mindful Eating**: Mindful eating involves paying attention to the food you eat, savoring each bite, and recognizing hunger and fullness cues. This practice can help improve digestion, enhance the enjoyment of food, and promote a healthy relationship with eating.

10. **Regular Medical Check-Ups**: Regular follow-ups with healthcare providers are essential for monitoring health, managing treatment side effects, and addressing any concerns. Staying informed and proactive about your health can lead to better outcomes.

PART I: GETTING STARTED

Preparing Your Healing Kitchen

Creating a healing kitchen is an essential step for anyone looking to support their health through nutrition, especially for cancer patients. A well-organized kitchen stocked with the right tools, ingredients, and knowledge can make meal preparation easier and more enjoyable. "The Great Cancer Diet Cookbook: Healing Recipes and Meal Plans for Cancer Patients" provides practical guidance on how to set up your kitchen for success. This article will cover essential kitchen tools and gadgets, how to stock your pantry with cancer-fighting foods, grocery shopping tips, and how to read and understand food labels.

Essential Kitchen Tools and Gadgets

Equipping your kitchen with the right tools and gadgets can significantly streamline the cooking process, making it easier to prepare nutritious meals that support cancer treatment and recovery. Here are some must-have items:

1. **Quality Chef's Knife**: A sharp, durable chef's knife is indispensable for chopping vegetables, fruits, and proteins. It makes meal prep faster and safer.

2. **Cutting Boards**: Have at least two cutting boards—one for produce and one for meat—to prevent cross-contamination. Bamboo or plastic cutting boards are easy to clean and maintain.

3. **Blender**: A high-speed blender is perfect for making smoothies, soups, and sauces. Look for one that can handle both liquids and solids efficiently.

4. **Food Processor**: This versatile tool can chop, slice, and puree ingredients, saving you time and effort in the kitchen. It's great for making dips, dressings, and finely chopped veggies.

5. **Slow Cooker or Instant Pot**: These appliances are ideal for preparing nutrient-dense meals with minimal effort. They can cook soups, stews, and casseroles while you focus on other tasks.

6. **Steamer Basket**: Steaming is one of the healthiest ways to cook vegetables, preserving their nutrients and flavor. A steamer basket fits into most pots and is easy to use.

7. **Non-Toxic Cookware**: Invest in high-quality, non-toxic cookware such as stainless steel, cast iron, or ceramic. Avoid non-stick pans with harmful coatings that can leach chemicals into your food.

8. **Measuring Cups and Spoons**: Accurate measurements are crucial for following recipes, especially when adjusting portion sizes or nutritional content.

9. **Digital Kitchen Scale**: This tool helps with portion control and ensures you're using the right amount of ingredients, which is

particularly important for managing dietary needs.

10. **Storage Containers**: Keep your pantry and fridge organized with a variety of airtight containers. Glass containers are preferred for storing leftovers and meal prep items.

11. **Salad Spinner**: This gadget makes washing and drying leafy greens quick and easy, which is essential for preparing fresh salads.

12. **Microplane or Zester**: Useful for grating citrus zest, garlic, and ginger, adding fresh flavors to your dishes without extra calories or salt.

Stocking Your Pantry with Cancer-Fighting Foods

A well-stocked pantry is the foundation of a healing kitchen. Keeping essential cancer-fighting foods on hand ensures that you always have the ingredients needed to prepare nutritious meals. Here are key categories and specific items to include:

1. **Whole Grains**:
   - Brown rice
   - Quinoa
   - Barley
   - Oats
   - Whole wheat pasta

2. **Legumes**:
   - Lentils
   - Chickpeas
   - Black beans
   - Kidney beans
   - Split peas

3. **Nuts and Seeds**:
   - Almonds
   - Walnuts
   - Chia seeds
   - Flaxseeds
   - Pumpkin seeds

4. **Healthy Oils and Fats**:
   - Extra virgin olive oil
   - Coconut oil
   - Avocado oil

- Nut butters (almond, peanut, cashew)

5. Dried Herbs and Spices:
  - Turmeric
  - Ginger
  - Garlic powder
  - Oregano
  - Thyme
  - Cumin
  - Cinnamon

6. Canned Goods:
  - Diced tomatoes (BPA-free cans or glass jars)
  - Coconut milk
  - Vegetable broth
  - Low-sodium beans

7. Condiments:
  - Apple cider vinegar
  - Balsamic vinegar
  - Tamari or low-sodium soy sauce
  - Dijon mustard
  - Nutritional yeast

8. **Baking Essentials:**
   - Whole wheat flour
   - Almond flour
   - Baking soda
   - Baking powder
   - Raw cacao powder

9. **Superfoods:**
   - Goji berries
   - Raw cacao nibs
   - Spirulina or chlorella powder
   - Matcha green tea powder

10. **Snack Items:**
    - Unsweetened dried fruit (apricots, figs, raisins)
    - Seaweed snacks
    - Whole grain crackers
    - Dark chocolate (70% cocoa or higher)

Grocery Shopping Tips for Cancer Patients

Grocery shopping can be overwhelming, especially when dealing with cancer treatment and its side effects. Here are some tips to make your shopping trips more efficient and less stressful:

1. **Plan Ahead**: Create a weekly meal plan and make a detailed shopping list before heading to the store. This helps you stay focused and avoid impulse purchases.

2. **Shop the Perimeter:** The outer aisles of the grocery store typically contain fresh produce, meats, dairy, and whole grains. Focus on these sections to find the most nutritious options.

3. **Buy Organic When Possible**: Organic produce is free from pesticides and other chemicals that can be harmful. Prioritize organic options for the "Dirty Dozen" (foods with the highest pesticide residues).

4. **Choose Fresh and Seasonal**: Fresh, seasonal produce is often more nutritious and flavorful. It can also be more cost-effective than out-of-season items.

5. **Read Labels**: Take the time to read food labels and ingredient lists. Look for products

with minimal ingredients and avoid those with added sugars, artificial additives, and high sodium levels.

6. **Consider Convenience**: If energy levels are low, consider pre-washed and pre-cut fruits and vegetables. Frozen produce is also a great option, as it retains its nutritional value and can be easily added to meals.

7. **Bulk Buying**: Purchase staple items like grains, legumes, nuts, and seeds in bulk to save money and reduce packaging waste. Store them in airtight containers to maintain freshness.

8. **Shop Local:** Support local farmers and markets for fresh, sustainably grown produce. Local foods are often fresher and have a smaller carbon footprint.

9. **Budget-Friendly Options**: If cost is a concern, prioritize nutrient-dense foods like beans, lentils, whole grains, and frozen vegetables. These items are affordable and versatile.

10. **Stay Hydrated**: Bring a water bottle with you to stay hydrated while shopping. Proper hydration can help maintain energy levels and reduce fatigue.

Reading and Understanding Food Labels

Understanding food labels is crucial for making informed choices that support your health. Here's a breakdown of key components to look for on food labels:

1. **Ingredients List:**

- Short and Simple: Choose products with a short, simple ingredient list. The fewer ingredients, the better.

- Whole Foods: Look for whole food ingredients rather than processed ones. Ingredients should be recognizable and pronounceable.

- Order of Ingredients: Ingredients are listed in order of quantity, from highest to lowest. The first few ingredients are the most significant.

2. **Nutrition Facts Panel:**

- Serving Size: Check the serving size and the number of servings per container. This helps you understand the nutritional content for the amount you're actually consuming.

- Calories: Be mindful of calorie content, especially if you need to manage your weight.

- Macronutrients: Look at the amounts of total fat, saturated fat, trans fat, cholesterol, sodium, total carbohydrates, dietary fiber, sugars, and protein. Aim for products with high fiber, low sugar, and healthy fats.

- Vitamins and Minerals: Check for vitamins and minerals like vitamin D, calcium, iron, and potassium. These nutrients are important for overall health.

3. **Specific Nutrients to Watch:**

- Added Sugars: Aim to minimize added sugars in your diet. Look for labels that specify "no added sugars" or have low amounts.

- Sodium: High sodium intake can lead to high blood pressure and other health issues. Choose low-sodium or no-salt-added products whenever possible.

- Fats: Focus on products with healthy fats (unsaturated fats) and avoid trans fats. Limit saturated fats to reduce the risk of heart disease.

4. Claims and Certifications:

- Organic: USDA Organic certification ensures that the product is free from synthetic pesticides, herbicides, and GMOs.
- Non-GMO: The Non-GMO Project Verified seal indicates that the product is free from genetically modified organisms.
- Whole Grain: Products with the Whole Grain Stamp contain significant amounts of whole grains.
- Low-Fat/Low-Sugar: Be cautious of "low-fat" or "low-sugar" claims. These products may contain added sugars or artificial ingredients to compensate for flavor.

5. Hidden Ingredients:

- Artificial Additives: Avoid artificial colors, flavors, and preservatives. These can contribute to health issues and may not be necessary for a nutritious diet.

- Sweeteners: Be aware of different names for added sugars, such as high fructose corn syrup, cane sugar, agave nectar, and molasses. Also, watch for artificial sweeteners like aspartame and sucralose.

Preparing a healing kitchen involves more than just cooking; it's about creating an environment that supports health and well-being through thoughtful planning and organization. By equipping your kitchen with essential tools and gadgets, stocking it with cancer-fighting foods, shopping wisely, and understanding food labels, you can make nutritious meal preparation a seamless part of your daily routine. "The Great Cancer Diet Cookbook: Healing Recipes and Meal Plans for Cancer Patients" is designed to guide you through each step, providing practical advice and delicious recipes that nourish the body and support recovery. With the right resources and knowledge, you can take an active role in your health journey and make every meal a step towards healing.

Nutrition Basics for Cancer Patients

Cancer patients face unique nutritional challenges that require careful attention to their diet. Proper nutrition can play a significant role in both cancer prevention and recovery, aiding in the body's ability to heal and withstand treatment. "The Great Cancer Diet Cookbook: Healing Recipes and Meal Plans for Cancer Patients" provides comprehensive guidance on how to meet these nutritional needs effectively. This article delves into key nutrients necessary for cancer patients, addresses common nutritional challenges during treatment, and offers long-term strategies for maintaining health post-treatment.

Key Nutrients for Cancer Prevention and Recovery

A balanced diet rich in specific nutrients is essential for cancer patients. These nutrients support the immune system, promote healing, and may even help prevent cancer recurrence.

Vitamins and Minerals

1. Vitamin C:
   - Role: Enhances immune function, aids in tissue repair, and acts as an antioxidant to protect cells from damage.
   - Sources: Citrus fruits, strawberries, bell peppers, broccoli, and Brussels sprouts.

2. Vitamin D:
   - Role: Crucial for bone health and immune regulation.
   - Sources: Sunlight exposure, fatty fish (salmon, mackerel), fortified dairy products, and egg yolks.

3. Vitamin E:
   - Role: Acts as an antioxidant, protecting cells from oxidative stress.
   - Sources: Nuts, seeds, spinach, broccoli, and sunflower oil.

4. Vitamin A:
   - Role: Important for immune function, vision, and cellular communication.
   - Sources: Carrots, sweet potatoes, dark leafy greens, and liver.

5. B Vitamins (B6, B12, Folate):
   - Role: Essential for energy production, DNA synthesis, and maintaining healthy nerve cells.
   - Sources: Whole grains, legumes, nuts, seeds, meat, eggs, and dairy products.

6. Calcium:
   - Role: Necessary for bone health and muscle function.
   - Sources: Dairy products, fortified plant milks, leafy greens, almonds, and tofu.

7. Iron:
   - Role: Vital for oxygen transport in the blood, preventing anemia and fatigue.
   - Sources: Lean meats, beans, lentils, spinach, and fortified cereals.

8. Zinc:
- Role: Supports immune function and wound healing.
- Sources: Meat, shellfish, legumes, seeds, nuts, and whole grains.

Phytochemicals and Antioxidants

Phytochemicals are compounds found in plants that have protective effects against cancer. Antioxidants help to neutralize free radicals, which can damage cells and lead to cancer.

1. Flavonoids:
- Role: Have anti-inflammatory and antioxidant properties.
- Sources: Berries, apples, onions, and green tea.

2. Carotenoids:
- Role: Protect cells from damage and enhance immune function.
- Sources: Carrots, sweet potatoes, spinach, and kale.

3. Sulforaphane:
   - Role: May help protect against cancer by enhancing detoxification enzymes.
   - Sources: Broccoli, Brussels sprouts, and cauliflower.

4. Lycopene:
   - Role: Associated with a reduced risk of certain cancers.
   - Sources: Tomatoes, watermelon, and pink grapefruit.

5. Polyphenols:
   - Role: Have antioxidant and anti-inflammatory effects.
   - Sources: Tea, coffee, red wine, grapes, and dark chocolate.

Protein, Carbohydrates, and Fats

A balanced intake of macronutrients is crucial for maintaining energy levels, supporting immune function, and aiding in recovery.

1. Protein:
   - Role: Essential for tissue repair, immune function, and maintaining muscle mass.
   - Sources: Lean meats, poultry, fish, eggs, dairy products, legumes, nuts, and seeds.

2. Carbohydrates:
   - Role: Provide energy and support brain function. Focus on complex carbohydrates for sustained energy.
   - Sources: Whole grains, fruits, vegetables, legumes, and oats.

3. Fats:
   - Role: Necessary for hormone production, brain function, and absorption of fat-soluble vitamins (A, D, E, K).
   - Sources: Avocado, nuts, seeds, olive oil, and fatty fish.

Addressing Nutritional Challenges During Treatment

Cancer treatments such as chemotherapy and radiation can lead to various side effects that impact nutritional intake. Managing these challenges effectively is crucial for maintaining health and strength during treatment.

Managing Appetite Changes

1. Small, Frequent Meals: Eating smaller, more frequent meals can help manage reduced appetite and ensure adequate calorie intake.
2. Nutrient-Dense Foods: Focus on foods that are high in calories and nutrients to maximize intake when appetite is low.
3. Appetite Stimulants: Using herbs and spices to enhance flavor and stimulate appetite can be beneficial.
4. Hydration: Staying hydrated is important, but avoid filling up on liquids before meals to prevent feeling too full.

Coping with Treatment Side Effects

1. Nausea and Vomiting:
   - Tips: Eat small, bland meals and avoid strong odors. Ginger tea and peppermint can help soothe nausea.

- Foods: Crackers, toast, bananas, and clear broths.

2. Mouth Sores and Difficulty Swallowing:
   - Tips: Choose soft, moist foods and avoid acidic or spicy items. Cold foods may be more soothing.
   - Foods: Smoothies, yogurt, mashed potatoes, and soft fruits.

3. Diarrhea:
   - Tips: Stay hydrated, avoid high-fiber foods, and eat small, frequent meals.
   - Foods: Bananas, rice, applesauce, and toast (BRAT diet).

4. Constipation:
   - Tips: Increase fiber intake, stay hydrated, and engage in light physical activity.
   - Foods: Whole grains, fruits, vegetables, and plenty of water.

5. Taste Changes:
   - Tips: Experiment with different flavors, seasonings, and textures. Cold foods may taste better than hot ones.

- Foods: Citrus fruits, flavored water, and marinated proteins.

Long-Term Nutritional Strategies for Survivors

Post-treatment nutrition is vital for maintaining health, preventing recurrence, and supporting overall well-being. Adopting sustainable dietary habits can lead to long-term benefits.

Maintaining a Balanced Diet Post-Treatment

1. Variety: Eat a wide range of foods to ensure you're getting a variety of nutrients. Incorporate different colors, textures, and flavors into your meals.
2. Whole Foods: Focus on whole, minimally processed foods. These are typically higher in nutrients and lower in added sugars, fats, and sodium.
3. Portion Control: Be mindful of portion sizes to maintain a healthy weight. Use smaller plates and serve reasonable portions.

4. Regular Meals: Establish a routine of regular meals and snacks to keep energy levels stable and avoid overeating.

Foods to Support Overall Health

1. Leafy Greens: Rich in vitamins, minerals, and fiber, leafy greens like spinach, kale, and Swiss chard are excellent for overall health.
2. Berries: Packed with antioxidants, berries such as blueberries, strawberries, and raspberries can help protect against oxidative stress.
3. Nuts and Seeds: Sources of healthy fats, protein, and fiber, nuts and seeds support heart health and provide sustained energy.
4. Whole Grains: Whole grains like quinoa, brown rice, and oats provide fiber, B vitamins, and other essential nutrients.
5. Lean Proteins: Lean proteins such as chicken, turkey, fish, and plant-based options like tofu and legumes are crucial for muscle repair and immune function.
6. Healthy Fats: Incorporate sources of healthy fats like avocados, olive oil, and fatty

fish to support brain health and hormone production.

7. Fermented Foods: Foods like yogurt, kefir, sauerkraut, and kimchi promote gut health by providing beneficial probiotics.

8. Hydration: Ensure adequate hydration by drinking water, herbal teas, and consuming water-rich fruits and vegetables.

Proper nutrition is a cornerstone of cancer prevention, treatment, and recovery. By focusing on key nutrients, managing the challenges that arise during treatment, and adopting long-term healthy eating habits, cancer patients can support their body's healing processes and improve their overall quality of life. "The Great Cancer Diet Cookbook: Healing Recipes and Meal Plans for Cancer Patients" offers practical advice and delicious recipes to help you navigate your nutritional journey, empowering you to take an active role in your health and well-being.

Meal Planning and Preparation

Meal planning and preparation are essential components of a healthy diet, especially for cancer patients. "The Great Cancer Diet Cookbook: Healing Recipes and Meal Plans for Cancer Patients" offers practical guidance on creating personalized meal plans, efficient meal prep techniques, and budget-friendly strategies to support individuals through their cancer journey.

Creating Personalized Meal Plans

Personalized meal plans are tailored to meet the specific nutritional needs and preferences of each individual. They ensure a well-balanced diet that supports overall health and well-being during cancer treatment and recovery.

Weekly Meal Planning Templates

1. Assess Nutritional Needs: Begin by assessing your nutritional needs based on

factors such as age, gender, weight, activity level, and any dietary restrictions or preferences.

2. Plan Balanced Meals: Use a weekly meal planning template to map out breakfast, lunch, dinner, and snacks for each day. Include a variety of nutrient-rich foods from all food groups.

3. Incorporate Cancer-Fighting Foods: Prioritize foods known for their cancer-fighting properties, such as fruits, vegetables, whole grains, lean proteins, and healthy fats.

4. Consider Treatment Side Effects: Take into account any treatment side effects that may affect appetite, taste preferences, or digestion. Adjust meal plans accordingly to accommodate these challenges.

5. Seek Variety: Aim for variety in your meals to ensure you're getting a wide range of nutrients. Experiment with different flavors, cuisines, and cooking methods to keep meals interesting.

Adjusting Plans for Individual Needs

1. Consult with Healthcare Team: Consult with your healthcare team, including a registered dietitian, to develop a meal plan that meets your individual needs and addresses any specific dietary concerns.

2. Monitor Progress: Monitor your progress and make adjustments to your meal plan as needed based on changes in appetite, weight, energy levels, and treatment side effects.

3. Flexibility: Be flexible with your meal plan and allow room for changes based on how you're feeling. Listen to your body and adjust your meals accordingly to ensure you're getting the nourishment you need.

Efficient Meal Prep Techniques

Efficient meal prep techniques help save time and energy in the kitchen, making it easier to stick to a healthy eating plan, even during busy or challenging times.

Time-Saving Tips

1. Plan Ahead: Set aside time each week to plan your meals, create a shopping list, and prep ingredients in advance. Having a plan in place reduces decision fatigue and makes mealtime less stressful.

2. Use Shortcuts: Take advantage of pre-cut vegetables, pre-cooked grains, and canned beans to streamline meal prep. These convenience items can save valuable time without sacrificing nutrition.

3. Multi-Task: Maximize efficiency by multitasking during meal prep. For example, while vegetables are roasting in the oven, you can prepare a salad or cook grains on the stovetop.

4. One-Pot Meals: Simplify cleanup and save time by cooking one-pot meals such as soups, stews, and casseroles. These dishes can be made in large batches and enjoyed throughout the week.

Batch Cooking and Freezing

1. Cook in Batches: Batch cooking involves preparing large quantities of food at once, which can then be portioned out and stored for future meals. This approach saves time and ensures you always have healthy options on hand.

2. Freeze Extra Portions: Invest in freezer-safe containers and freeze extra portions of meals for later use. Label containers with the date and contents for easy identification.

3. Meal Prep Sessions: Dedicate a day each week to a meal prep session where you can cook, portion, and package meals for the week ahead. This proactive approach simplifies mealtime and reduces the temptation to reach for unhealthy convenience foods.

4. Freezer-Friendly Foods: Certain foods freeze well and can be easily reheated for quick meals. Examples include soups, stews, chili, casseroles, cooked grains, and homemade sauces.

Budget-Friendly Meal Planning

Eating healthy on a budget is possible with careful planning and smart shopping strategies. "The Great Cancer Diet Cookbook: Healing Recipes and Meal Plans for Cancer Patients" provides budget-friendly meal planning tips to make nutritious eating accessible to everyone.

Affordable Cancer-Fighting Foods

1. Buy in Bulk: Purchase staple items like grains, legumes, nuts, and seeds in bulk to save money. These ingredients are versatile and can be used in a variety of recipes.
2. Seasonal Produce: Shop for seasonal fruits and vegetables, as they tend to be more affordable and flavorful. Visit farmers' markets or join a community-supported agriculture (CSA) program for fresh, locally grown produce.
3. Frozen Fruits and Vegetables: Frozen fruits and vegetables are often more affordable than fresh and have the added benefit of a longer

shelf life. Use them in smoothies, stir-fries, soups, and casseroles.

4. Plant-Based Proteins: Incorporate plant-based proteins such as beans, lentils, tofu, and tempeh into your meals. These options are generally less expensive than animal proteins and offer similar nutritional benefits.

5. Limit Processed Foods: Minimize spending on processed and convenience foods, which tend to be more expensive and less nutritious. Focus on whole, minimally processed foods that provide maximum nutrition for your dollar.

Shopping on a Budget

1. Plan Your Meals: Create a meal plan and shopping list based on budget-friendly recipes and seasonal ingredients. Stick to your list to avoid impulse purchases.

2. Compare Prices: Compare prices between different brands and stores to find the best deals on essential items. Consider purchasing store brands or generic equivalents to save money.

3. Shop Sales and Discounts: Take advantage of sales, discounts, and coupons to lower your grocery bill. Stock up on non-perishable items when they're on sale and freeze extras for later use.

4. Avoid Waste: Minimize food waste by using leftovers creatively, repurposing ingredients in multiple meals, and storing perishable items properly to extend their shelf life.

5. Grow Your Own: Consider growing your own herbs, fruits, and vegetables if space allows. Gardening can be a cost-effective way to access fresh produce and connect with nature.

Meal planning and preparation are essential skills for cancer patients looking to optimize their nutrition and support their overall health during treatment and recovery. By creating personalized meal plans, utilizing efficient meal prep techniques, and implementing budget-friendly strategies, individuals can ensure they're getting the nourishment they need without breaking the bank. "The Great Cancer Diet Cookbook: Healing Recipes and Meal Plans for Cancer

Patients" provides practical guidance and delicious recipes to empower individuals on their journey to wellness, making healthy eating accessible and enjoyable for all.

PART II: HEALING RECIPES FOR EVERY MEAL

Breakfast Recipes for Cancer Patients

Starting your day with a nutritious breakfast is essential for fueling your body and providing the energy you need to tackle the day ahead. These breakfast recipes from "The Great Cancer Diet Cookbook" are not only delicious but also packed with cancer-fighting nutrients to support your health and well-being during treatment and recovery.

Energizing Smoothies and Juices

Smoothies and juices are a quick and convenient way to pack in a variety of nutrients, making them an ideal choice for busy mornings. These recipes are designed to provide a burst of energy and nourishment to kick-start your day.

Green Power Smoothie

Ingredients:
- 1 cup spinach leaves
- 1/2 cup kale leaves, stemmed

- 1/2 cup cucumber, chopped
- 1/2 cup frozen pineapple chunks
- 1/2 banana
- 1 tablespoon chia seeds
- 1 cup coconut water or almond milk
- Ice cubes (optional)

Cooking Instructions:
1. Place spinach, kale, cucumber, pineapple chunks, banana, chia seeds, and coconut water (or almond milk) in a blender.
2. Blend on high until smooth and creamy. Add ice cubes if desired for a colder consistency.
3. Pour into a glass and serve immediately.

Cook Tips:
- Customize your smoothie by adding other fruits such as mango, berries, or apple for extra flavor and nutrients.
- For added protein, incorporate a scoop of protein powder or Greek yogurt into the smoothie.

Nutritional Value:
- This green power smoothie is rich in vitamins, minerals, and antioxidants. Spinach and kale provide a healthy dose of vitamin K, vitamin A, and folate, while pineapple adds sweetness and vitamin C. Chia seeds offer omega-3 fatty acids and fiber, making this smoothie a nutritious way to start your day.

Berry Antioxidant Smoothie

Ingredients:
- 1/2 cup mixed berries (such as strawberries, blueberries, and raspberries)
- 1/2 banana
- 1/2 cup plain Greek yogurt
- 1 tablespoon honey or maple syrup (optional)
- 1/2 cup almond milk or coconut water
- Ice cubes (optional)

Cooking Instructions:
1. Combine mixed berries, banana, Greek yogurt, honey or maple syrup (if using), and almond milk (or coconut water) in a blender.

2. Blend on high until smooth and creamy. Add ice cubes if desired for a thicker consistency.

3. Pour into a glass and garnish with additional berries if desired. Serve immediately.

Cook Tips:

- Use frozen berries for a colder and thicker smoothie.

- Adjust sweetness by adding more or less honey or maple syrup according to your taste preferences.

Nutritional Value:

- This berry antioxidant smoothie is packed with vitamins, antioxidants, and probiotics. Berries are rich in antioxidants such as anthocyanins, which help fight inflammation and oxidative stress. Greek yogurt provides probiotics for gut health, while banana adds potassium and natural sweetness. Enjoy this refreshing smoothie as a delicious and nutritious way to start your day.

Nutritious Breakfast Bowls

Breakfast bowls offer a customizable and satisfying option for a wholesome morning meal. These recipes feature nourishing ingredients like quinoa, oats, nuts, and seeds to provide sustained energy and support your health goals.

Quinoa and Berry Breakfast Bowl

Ingredients:
- 1/2 cup cooked quinoa
- 1/2 cup mixed berries (such as strawberries, blueberries, and raspberries)
- 2 tablespoons chopped nuts (such as almonds, walnuts, or pecans)
- 1 tablespoon chia seeds or flaxseeds
- 1 tablespoon honey or maple syrup (optional)
- 1/4 cup plain Greek yogurt or almond milk

Cooking Instructions:
1. In a bowl, layer cooked quinoa, mixed berries, chopped nuts, and chia seeds or flaxseeds.

2. Drizzle with honey or maple syrup (if using) for added sweetness.

3. Serve with a dollop of plain Greek yogurt or almond milk on top.

Cook Tips:

- Cook quinoa ahead of time and store it in the refrigerator for quick and easy assembly in the morning.

- Customize your breakfast bowl by adding other toppings such as sliced bananas, shredded coconut, or granola for extra texture and flavor.

Nutritional Value:

- This quinoa and berry breakfast bowl is a nutrient-packed meal that provides a balance of carbohydrates, protein, fiber, and healthy fats. Quinoa is a complete protein, meaning it contains all nine essential amino acids, making it an excellent choice for vegetarians and vegans. Berries are rich in antioxidants, while nuts and seeds offer heart-healthy fats and essential nutrients. Enjoy this satisfying breakfast bowl for sustained energy and a nutritious start to your day.

Oatmeal with Nuts and Seeds

Ingredients:
- 1/2 cup rolled oats
- 1 cup water or milk (dairy or plant-based)
- 1/4 teaspoon ground cinnamon
- 1 tablespoon chopped nuts (such as almonds, walnuts, or pecans)
- 1 tablespoon seeds (such as chia seeds, flaxseeds, or pumpkin seeds)
- 1 tablespoon honey or maple syrup (optional)
- Fresh fruit for topping (such as sliced bananas, berries, or apple slices)

Cooking Instructions:
1. In a small saucepan, bring water or milk to a boil. Stir in rolled oats and reduce heat to low.
2. Cook, stirring occasionally, for 5-7 minutes or until oats are creamy and tender.
3. Remove from heat and stir in ground cinnamon, chopped nuts, seeds, and honey or maple syrup (if using).
4. Transfer oatmeal to a bowl and top with fresh fruit of your choice.

Cook Tips:
- Experiment with different toppings and flavor combinations, such as adding nut butter, dried fruit, or shredded coconut.
- To save time in the morning, prepare a batch of oatmeal ahead of time and reheat individual servings as needed.

Nutritional Value:
- Oatmeal with nuts and seeds is a nutritious and comforting breakfast option that provides a balance of complex carbohydrates, protein, fiber, and essential nutrients. Oats are a good source of soluble fiber, which helps lower cholesterol levels and promotes heart health. Nuts and seeds add healthy fats, protein, and additional fiber, while cinnamon offers anti-inflammatory properties. Enjoy this hearty breakfast to fuel your body and start your day on a nutritious note.

Easy Breakfast Recipes

Breakfast is often considered the most important meal of the day, especially for cancer patients undergoing treatment. These easy breakfast recipes from "The Great Cancer Diet Cookbook" are designed to provide nourishment, energy, and delicious flavors to support your health and well-being during your cancer journey.

Chia Seed Pudding

Chia seed pudding is a nutritious and versatile breakfast option that can be customized with your favorite toppings and flavors. Rich in fiber, protein, and omega-3 fatty acids, chia seeds offer a variety of health benefits, including improved digestion, heart health, and energy levels. This recipe is easy to prepare and can be made ahead of time for a convenient grab-and-go breakfast option.

Ingredients:
- 1/4 cup chia seeds
- 1 cup almond milk or coconut milk
- 1 tablespoon maple syrup or honey (optional)
- 1/2 teaspoon vanilla extract

- Fresh fruit, nuts, seeds, or granola for topping (optional)

Cooking Instructions:
1. In a mixing bowl or jar, combine chia seeds, almond milk (or coconut milk), maple syrup or honey (if using), and vanilla extract. Stir well to combine.
2. Cover the bowl or jar and refrigerate for at least 4 hours or overnight to allow the chia seeds to absorb the liquid and thicken into a pudding-like consistency.
3. Once the chia seed pudding has set, stir well to break up any clumps and adjust the sweetness to taste, if necessary.
4. Serve the chia seed pudding in individual bowls or jars and top with your favorite toppings, such as fresh fruit, nuts, seeds, or granola.
5. Enjoy immediately or store any leftovers in an airtight container in the refrigerator for up to 3 days.

Cook Tips:
- Experiment with different flavors by adding ingredients such as cocoa powder, cinnamon,

or matcha powder to the chia seed mixture before refrigerating.

- Customize your chia seed pudding with a variety of toppings, such as sliced bananas, berries, chopped nuts, shredded coconut, or dried fruit.

- For a creamier texture, blend the chia seed pudding mixture in a blender before refrigerating to break up the chia seeds and create a smoother consistency.

Nutritional Value:
- Chia seeds are a nutritional powerhouse, packed with fiber, protein, omega-3 fatty acids, and antioxidants. They provide sustained energy, promote satiety, and support digestive health. Almond milk or coconut milk adds additional nutrients such as calcium, vitamin D, and healthy fats. Enjoy this nutrient-rich chia seed pudding as a satisfying and nourishing breakfast option to start your day on the right foot.

Whole Grain Pancakes with Fruit Compote

Whole grain pancakes with fruit compote are a comforting and wholesome breakfast option that's perfect for special occasions or leisurely weekend mornings. Made with whole grain flour, these pancakes are rich in fiber, vitamins, and minerals, providing sustained energy and supporting overall health. The fruit compote adds natural sweetness and a burst of flavor, making this breakfast both delicious and nutritious.

Ingredients:
- 1 cup whole wheat flour or whole grain pancake mix
- 1 tablespoon sugar or maple syrup (optional)
- 1 teaspoon baking powder
- 1/2 teaspoon baking soda
- 1/4 teaspoon salt
- 1 cup buttermilk or almond milk
- 1 egg
- 2 tablespoons melted butter or coconut oil
- 1 teaspoon vanilla extract
- Fresh fruit (such as berries, sliced bananas, or chopped apples) for topping

For the Fruit Compote:
- 1 cup fresh or frozen fruit (such as berries, peaches, or cherries)
- 1 tablespoon honey or maple syrup
- 1 tablespoon water
- 1/2 teaspoon lemon juice
- 1/4 teaspoon vanilla extract
- Pinch of cinnamon (optional)

Cooking Instructions:
1. In a mixing bowl, whisk together whole wheat flour or pancake mix, sugar or maple syrup (if using), baking powder, baking soda, and salt.
2. In a separate bowl, whisk together buttermilk or almond milk, egg, melted butter or coconut oil, and vanilla extract.
3. Pour the wet ingredients into the dry ingredients and stir until just combined. Be careful not to overmix; the batter should be slightly lumpy.
4. Heat a non-stick skillet or griddle over medium heat and lightly grease with cooking spray or additional butter.

5. Pour 1/4 cup of batter onto the skillet for each pancake and cook until bubbles form on the surface, then flip and cook until golden brown on both sides. Repeat with the remaining batter.

6. While the pancakes are cooking, prepare the fruit compote. In a small saucepan, combine fresh or frozen fruit, honey or maple syrup, water, lemon juice, vanilla extract, and cinnamon (if using). Bring to a simmer over medium heat and cook for 5-7 minutes, or until the fruit is soft and the sauce has thickened slightly.

7. Serve the pancakes warm with the fruit compote drizzled on top. Garnish with additional fresh fruit if desired.

Cook Tips:

- For lighter and fluffier pancakes, separate the egg and beat the egg white until stiff peaks form, then fold it into the batter just before cooking.

- Make a double batch of pancakes and freeze the extras for later use. Simply place cooled pancakes in a single layer on a baking sheet

and freeze until firm, then transfer to a resealable plastic bag or container for storage.
- Experiment with different fruit combinations for the compote, such as mixed berries, peaches and raspberries, or cherries and plums.

Nutritional Value:
- Whole grain pancakes provide a good source of complex carbohydrates, fiber, and essential nutrients such as B vitamins, iron, and magnesium. The fruit compote adds natural sweetness and additional vitamins, minerals, and antioxidants. Enjoy this delicious and nutritious breakfast option as a satisfying way to start your day on a wholesome note.

Lunch Recipes for Cancer Patients

Lunch is an important meal that provides the opportunity to refuel and nourish your body midday. These lunch recipes from "The Great Cancer Diet Cookbook" are designed to be both satisfying and nutritious, offering a variety of options to suit different tastes and preferences.

Nourishing Salads

Salads are a versatile and refreshing lunch option that can be customized with a variety of ingredients to create a balanced and satisfying meal. Packed with vitamins, minerals, and fiber, these salads are designed to support your health and well-being during your cancer journey.

Kale and Quinoa Salad with Lemon Dressing

Ingredients:
- 2 cups kale leaves, stemmed and chopped
- 1 cup cooked quinoa, cooled

- 1/2 cup cherry tomatoes, halved
- 1/4 cup cucumber, diced
- 1/4 cup red onion, thinly sliced
- 1/4 cup feta cheese, crumbled (optional)
- 2 tablespoons sunflower seeds
- Lemon Dressing:
  - 2 tablespoons olive oil
  - 1 tablespoon fresh lemon juice
  - 1 teaspoon honey or maple syrup
  - 1/2 teaspoon Dijon mustard
  - Salt and pepper to taste

Cooking Instructions:
1. In a large mixing bowl, combine chopped kale, cooked quinoa, cherry tomatoes, cucumber, red onion, feta cheese (if using), and sunflower seeds.
2. In a small bowl, whisk together olive oil, lemon juice, honey or maple syrup, Dijon mustard, salt, and pepper to make the dressing.
3. Pour the dressing over the salad and toss until well coated.
4. Let the salad marinate for at least 10 minutes before serving to allow the flavors to meld together.

5. Divide the salad into individual bowls and serve as a light and nourishing lunch option.

Cook Tips:
- Massage the kale leaves with a small amount of olive oil before adding them to the salad to help soften their texture and reduce bitterness.
- Customize the salad by adding other vegetables such as bell peppers, carrots, or avocado, or incorporating additional protein sources such as grilled chicken, tofu, or chickpeas.

Nutritional Value:
- This kale and quinoa salad is rich in fiber, protein, vitamins, and minerals, making it a nutrient-dense meal that supports overall health and well-being. Kale is packed with antioxidants, vitamins A, C, and K, and calcium, while quinoa provides a complete source of protein and essential amino acids. Enjoy this refreshing salad as a satisfying and nourishing lunch option to fuel your body and satisfy your taste buds.

Spinach and Avocado Salad

Ingredients:
- 4 cups fresh spinach leaves
- 1 avocado, sliced
- 1/2 cup strawberries, sliced
- 1/4 cup red onion, thinly sliced
- 1/4 cup goat cheese, crumbled (optional)
- 2 tablespoons sliced almonds or pecans
- Balsamic Vinaigrette:
  - 2 tablespoons balsamic vinegar
  - 1 tablespoon olive oil
  - 1 teaspoon honey or maple syrup
  - Salt and pepper to taste

Cooking Instructions:
1. In a large salad bowl, combine fresh spinach leaves, sliced avocado, strawberries, red onion, goat cheese (if using), and sliced almonds or pecans.
2. In a small bowl, whisk together balsamic vinegar, olive oil, honey or maple syrup, salt, and pepper to make the vinaigrette.
3. Drizzle the vinaigrette over the salad and toss until well combined.

4. Serve the spinach and avocado salad immediately as a light and refreshing lunch option.

Cook Tips:
- Use ripe avocados for the best flavor and texture in the salad. Look for avocados that yield slightly to gentle pressure when squeezed.
- Toast the sliced almonds or pecans in a dry skillet over medium heat for a few minutes until golden brown and fragrant before adding them to the salad for extra crunch and flavor.

Nutritional Value:
- This spinach and avocado salad is packed with vitamins, minerals, antioxidants, and healthy fats, making it a nourishing and satisfying lunch option. Spinach is a good source of iron, vitamin C, and folate, while avocado provides heart-healthy monounsaturated fats and potassium. Enjoy this vibrant salad as a delicious and nutritious way to boost your intake of essential nutrients and support your overall health.

Hearty Soups and Stews

Soups and stews are comforting and nourishing lunch options that can be easily customized with a variety of ingredients to suit your taste preferences. These recipes are packed with vegetables, lean protein, and whole grains to provide sustained energy and support your health goals during your cancer journey.

Lentil and Vegetable Soup

Ingredients:
- 1 tablespoon olive oil
- 1 onion, chopped
- 2 carrots, diced
- 2 celery stalks, diced
- 2 garlic cloves, minced
- 1 cup dried green lentils, rinsed and drained
- 6 cups vegetable broth or chicken broth
- 1 can (14 ounces) diced tomatoes
- 2 bay leaves
- 1 teaspoon dried thyme
- Salt and pepper to taste
- Fresh parsley, chopped (for garnish)

Cooking Instructions:

1. In a large soup pot or Dutch oven, heat olive oil over medium heat. Add chopped onion, carrots, celery, and garlic, and sauté until softened, about 5 minutes.

2. Add dried lentils, vegetable broth or chicken broth, diced tomatoes (with juices), bay leaves, dried thyme, salt, and pepper to the pot. Stir to combine.

3. Bring the soup to a boil, then reduce heat to low and simmer, covered, for 25-30 minutes or until lentils are tender.

4. Remove the bay leaves from the soup and discard. Taste and adjust seasoning as needed.

5. Ladle the lentil and vegetable soup into individual bowls, garnish with chopped parsley, and serve hot.

Cook Tips:

- Customize the soup by adding other vegetables such as bell peppers, zucchini, or spinach, or incorporating additional protein sources such as diced chicken, turkey, or tofu.

- For added flavor, stir in a tablespoon of balsamic vinegar or a squeeze of lemon juice just before serving.

Nutritional Value:
- This lentil and vegetable soup is rich in fiber, protein, vitamins, and minerals, making it a nutritious and satisfying lunch option for cancer patients. Lentils are an excellent source of plant-based protein, fiber, iron, and folate, while vegetables provide vitamins A, C, and K, as well as antioxidants. Enjoy this hearty and flavorful soup as a comforting and nourishing meal to support your health and well-being.

Chicken and Barley Stew

Ingredients:
- 1 tablespoon olive oil
- 1 onion, chopped
- 2 carrots, diced
- 2 celery stalks, diced
- 2 garlic cloves, minced
- 1 pound boneless, skinless chicken breasts or thighs, cut into bite-sized pieces
- 1/2 cup pearl barley, rinsed and drained

- 6 cups chicken broth
- 1 can (14 ounces-) diced tomatoes
- 1 teaspoon dried thyme
- Salt and pepper to taste
- Fresh parsley, chopped (for garnish)

Cooking Instructions:

1. In a large soup pot or Dutch oven, heat olive oil over medium heat. Add chopped onion, carrots, celery, and garlic, and sauté until softened, about 5 minutes.

2. Add the diced chicken to the pot and cook until browned on all sides, about 5-7 minutes.

3. Stir in pearl barley, chicken broth, diced tomatoes (with juices), dried thyme, salt, and pepper.

4. Bring the stew to a boil, then reduce heat to low and simmer, covered, for 30-35 minutes or until the barley is tender and the chicken is cooked through.

5. Taste and adjust seasoning as needed. If the stew is too thick, you can add additional broth or water to reach your desired consistency.

6. Ladle the chicken and barley stew into individual bowls, garnish with chopped parsley, and serve hot.

Cook Tips:
- To save time, you can use pre-cooked chicken or rotisserie chicken and add it to the stew during the last 10 minutes of cooking.
- Feel free to add other vegetables such as potatoes, bell peppers, or green beans to the stew for added flavor and nutrition.

Nutritional Value:
- This chicken and barley stew is a hearty and nourishing meal that provides a balance of protein, carbohydrates, and fiber to support your health and well-being during your cancer journey. Chicken is a good source of lean protein, while barley offers fiber, vitamins, and minerals. Vegetables add essential nutrients and antioxidants to the stew, making it a nutritious and satisfying lunch option. Enjoy this comforting and flavorful stew as a delicious way to nourish your body and satisfy your appetite.

Filling Sandwiches and Wraps

Sandwiches and wraps are convenient and portable lunch options that can be packed with a variety of ingredients to create a balanced and satisfying meal. These recipes feature flavorful fillings and wholesome ingredients to provide energy and nourishment during your cancer journey.

Grilled Veggie Wrap with Hummus

Ingredients:
- 1 large whole wheat or spinach tortilla wrap
- 1/4 cup hummus
- 1/2 cup mixed grilled vegetables (such as bell peppers, zucchini, eggplant, and mushrooms), sliced
- 1/4 cup baby spinach leaves
- 2 tablespoons crumbled feta cheese (optional)
- 1 tablespoon chopped fresh herbs (such as parsley, basil, or cilantro)
- Salt and pepper to taste

Cooking Instructions:
1. Spread hummus evenly over the surface of the tortilla wrap.
2. Arrange grilled vegetables, baby spinach leaves, crumbled feta cheese (if using), and chopped fresh herbs on top of the hummus.
3. Season with salt and pepper to taste.
4. Roll up the tortilla wrap tightly, folding in the sides as you go, to create a compact wrap.
5. Slice the wrap in half diagonally and serve immediately, or wrap tightly in parchment paper or aluminum foil for later.

Cook Tips:
- Customize the wrap by using your favorite grilled vegetables or adding other ingredients such as avocado, roasted red peppers, or sun-dried tomatoes.
- To make the wrap gluten-free, use a gluten-free tortilla or wrap made from alternative grains such as brown rice or quinoa.

Nutritional Value:
- This grilled veggie wrap with hummus is a flavorful and satisfying lunch option that

provides a balance of carbohydrates, protein, and fiber to support your energy levels and overall health. Hummus offers plant-based protein and healthy fats, while grilled vegetables provide vitamins, minerals, and antioxidants. Enjoy this delicious and nutritious wrap as a convenient and portable meal during your busy day.

Hummus and Veggie Sandwich

Ingredients:
- 2 slices whole grain bread or gluten-free bread
- 1/4 cup hummus
- 1/2 cup mixed fresh vegetables (such as cucumber slices, tomato slices, shredded carrots, and lettuce leaves)
- 2 slices avocado
- Sprouts or microgreens for topping (optional)
- Salt and pepper to taste

Cooking Instructions:
1. Spread hummus evenly over one side of each slice of bread.

2. Layer mixed fresh vegetables, avocado slices, and sprouts or microgreens (if using) on top of one slice of bread.

3. Season with salt and pepper to taste.

4. Place the second slice of bread on top to form a sandwich.

5. Slice the sandwich in half diagonally and serve immediately, or wrap tightly in parchment paper or aluminum foil for later.

Cook Tips:
- Customize the sandwich by using your favorite vegetables or adding other ingredients such as roasted red peppers, grilled eggplant, or marinated artichoke hearts.
- For added protein, add slices of cooked chicken, turkey, tofu, or tempeh to the sandwich.

Nutritional Value:
- This hummus and veggie sandwich is a wholesome and satisfying lunch option that provides a variety of nutrients to support your health and well-being during your cancer journey. Whole grain bread offers fiber and

complex carbohydrates, while hummus provides plant-based protein and healthy fats. Fresh vegetables add vitamins, minerals, and antioxidants, making this sandwich a nutritious and delicious choice for lunch. Enjoy this flavorful and filling sandwich as a convenient and nourishing meal option.

Dinner Recipes for Cancer Patients

Dinner is an important meal that provides an opportunity to nourish your body with wholesome ingredients and balanced flavors. These dinner recipes from "The Great Cancer Diet Cookbook" are designed to be both delicious and nutritious, offering a variety of options to support your health and well-being during your cancer journey.

Balanced Main Courses

Balanced main courses are the cornerstone of a nutritious dinner, providing protein, healthy fats, and essential nutrients to support your health goals. These recipes feature flavorful and satisfying dishes that are easy to prepare and packed with wholesome ingredients.

Baked Salmon with Asparagus

Ingredients:
- 4 salmon fillets
- 1 bunch asparagus, trimmed

- 2 tablespoons olive oil
- 2 cloves garlic, minced
- 1 teaspoon lemon zest
- 1 tablespoon fresh lemon juice
- 1 teaspoon dried dill
- Salt and pepper to taste
- Lemon wedges for serving

Cooking Instructions:
1. Preheat the oven to 400°F (200°C). Line a baking sheet with parchment paper or aluminum foil.
2. Place the salmon fillets on the prepared baking sheet and arrange the asparagus around them.
3. In a small bowl, whisk together olive oil, minced garlic, lemon zest, lemon juice, dried dill, salt, and pepper.
4. Drizzle the olive oil mixture over the salmon and asparagus, ensuring that they are evenly coated.
5. Bake in the preheated oven for 12-15 minutes, or until the salmon is cooked through and the asparagus is tender.
6. Remove from the oven and serve immediately with lemon wedges on the side.

Cook Tips:
- Choose wild-caught salmon for its superior flavor and nutritional profile.
- To prevent overcooking, check the salmon for doneness after 10 minutes of baking. The fish should flake easily with a fork when done.

Nutritional Value:
- Salmon is rich in omega-3 fatty acids, protein, and vitamin D, making it an excellent choice for supporting heart health and reducing inflammation. Asparagus is a good source of fiber, vitamins A, C, and K, and folate, providing additional nutrients and flavor to this delicious main course.

Quinoa-Stuffed Bell Peppers

Ingredients:
- 4 large bell peppers, any color
- 1 cup quinoa, rinsed and drained
- 2 cups vegetable broth or chicken broth
- 1 tablespoon olive oil
- 1 onion, diced
- 2 cloves garlic, minced

- 1 zucchini, diced
- 1 carrot, diced
- 1 cup cherry tomatoes, halved
- 1/2 cup crumbled feta cheese (optional)
- 2 tablespoons chopped fresh parsley or basil
- Salt and pepper to taste

Cooking Instructions:
1. Preheat the oven to 375°F (190°C). Cut the tops off the bell peppers and remove the seeds and membranes.
2. In a medium saucepan, combine quinoa and vegetable broth or chicken broth. Bring to a boil, then reduce heat to low and simmer, covered, for 15-20 minutes or until the quinoa is cooked and the liquid is absorbed.
3. In a large skillet, heat olive oil over medium heat. Add diced onion and minced garlic, and sauté until softened, about 5 minutes.
4. Add diced zucchini and carrot to the skillet, and cook for an additional 5 minutes, or until vegetables are tender.
5. Remove the skillet from heat and stir in cooked quinoa, halved cherry tomatoes, crumbled feta cheese (if using), chopped fresh parsley or basil, salt, and pepper.

6. Spoon the quinoa mixture into the prepared bell peppers, pressing down gently to pack the filling.

7. Place the stuffed bell peppers upright in a baking dish, and cover loosely with aluminum foil.

8. Bake in the preheated oven for 25-30 minutes, or until the peppers are tender and the filling is heated through.

9. Remove from the oven and serve hot.

Cook Tips:

- Use any color of bell peppers for variety and visual appeal.

- Customize the filling by adding other vegetables such as corn, peas, or mushrooms, or incorporating additional protein sources such as cooked chicken, turkey, or tofu.

Nutritional Value:

- Quinoa is a gluten-free whole grain that is rich in protein, fiber, and essential amino acids, making it a nutritious and filling option for stuffed peppers. Combined with a variety of vegetables and optional feta cheese, this dish provides a balance of carbohydrates, protein, and vitamins to support your health and well-being during your cancer journey.

Plant-Based Proteins

Plant-based proteins are an excellent source of nutrition for cancer patients, offering protein, fiber, and essential nutrients without the saturated fat and cholesterol found in animal products. These recipes feature flavorful and satisfying plant-based dishes that are easy to prepare and packed with wholesome ingredients.

Chickpea and Spinach Curry

Ingredients:
- 2 tablespoons olive oil
- 1 onion, diced
- 3 cloves garlic, minced
- 1 tablespoon fresh ginger, grated
- 1 tablespoon curry powder
- 1 teaspoon ground cumin
- 1/2 teaspoon ground turmeric
- 1/4 teaspoon cayenne pepper (optional)

- 1 can (15 ounces) chickpeas, drained and rinsed
- 1 can (14 ounces) diced tomatoes
- 1 can (13.5 ounces) coconut milk
- 4 cups fresh spinach leaves
- Salt and pepper to taste
- Cooked rice or quinoa for serving

Cooking Instructions:
1. In a large skillet or saucepan, heat olive oil over medium heat. Add diced onion and sauté until softened, about 5 minutes.
2. Add minced garlic, grated ginger, curry powder, ground cumin, ground turmeric, and cayenne pepper (if using) to the skillet, and cook for an additional 2 minutes, stirring constantly.
3. Stir in drained chickpeas, diced tomatoes (with juices), and coconut milk, and bring to a simmer.
4. Reduce heat to low and simmer, uncovered, for 15-20 minutes, stirring occasionally, until the curry has thickened slightly.
5. Stir in fresh spinach leaves and cook for an additional 3-5 minutes, or until the spinach is wilted.

6. Season with salt and pepper to taste.
7. Serve the chickpea and spinach curry hot over cooked rice or quinoa.

Cook Tips:
- Customize the curry by adding other vegetables such as bell peppers, carrots, or cauliflower, or incorporating additional spices such as garam masala, coriander, or cinnamon.
- For a creamier texture, use full-fat coconut milk instead of light coconut milk.

Nutritional Value:
- Chickpeas are an excellent source of plant-based protein, fiber, and essential nutrients, making them a nutritious and filling ingredient for this curry. Combined with fresh spinach and aromatic spices, this dish offers a burst of flavor and nutrition that is sure to satisfy your taste buds while supporting your health and well-being during your cancer journey.

Black Bean and Sweet Potato Enchiladas

Ingredients:
- 1 tablespoon olive oil
- 1 onion, diced- 2 cloves garlic, minced
- 1 teaspoon ground cumin
- 1 teaspoon chili powder
- 1 can (15 ounces) black beans, drained and rinsed
- 1 large sweet potato, peeled and diced
- 1 cup frozen corn kernels
- 1 cup chopped spinach
- 1 cup enchilada sauce
- 8 whole wheat or corn tortillas
- 1 cup shredded cheese (cheddar or Monterey Jack), optional
- Fresh cilantro, chopped, for garnish
- Avocado slices, for serving (optional)

Cooking Instructions:
1. Preheat the oven to 375°F (190°C). Lightly grease a 9x13-inch baking dish.
2. In a large skillet, heat olive oil over medium heat. Add diced onion and minced garlic, and sauté until softened, about 5 minutes.

3. Add ground cumin and chili powder to the skillet, and cook for an additional 1-2 minutes, stirring constantly.

4. Stir in black beans, diced sweet potato, frozen corn kernels, chopped spinach, and 1/2 cup enchilada sauce. Cook for 8-10 minutes, or until the sweet potato is tender and the mixture is heated through.

5. Spread a thin layer of enchilada sauce on the bottom of the prepared baking dish.

6. Spoon the bean and sweet potato mixture onto each tortilla, and roll up tightly. Place the rolled enchiladas seam-side down in the baking dish.

7. Pour the remaining enchilada sauce over the top of the enchiladas, spreading evenly to cover.

8. If using, sprinkle shredded cheese over the top of the enchiladas.

9. Cover the baking dish with aluminum foil and bake in the preheated oven for 20-25 minutes, or until the enchiladas are heated through and the cheese is melted and bubbly.

10. Remove from the oven and garnish with chopped cilantro.

11. Serve the black bean and sweet potato enchiladas hot, with avocado slices on the side if desired.

Cook Tips:
- To save time, you can use canned or pre-cooked sweet potato instead of cooking it from scratch.
- Customize the enchiladas by adding other vegetables such as bell peppers, zucchini, or mushrooms, or incorporating additional protein sources such as tofu or shredded chicken.

Nutritional Value:
- Black beans are a rich source of plant-based protein, fiber, and essential nutrients, making them an excellent addition to these enchiladas. Combined with sweet potato, corn, spinach, and aromatic spices, this dish offers a balance of flavors and textures that is sure to satisfy your taste buds while providing essential nutrition to support your health and well-being during your cancer journey.

Healthy Side Dishes

Healthy side dishes complement your main course and provide additional nutrients and flavors to your meal. These recipes feature simple yet delicious side dishes that are easy to prepare and packed with wholesome ingredients.

Roasted Brussels Sprouts

Ingredients:
- 1 pound Brussels sprouts, trimmed and halved
- 2 tablespoons olive oil
- 2 cloves garlic, minced
- Salt and pepper to taste
- Grated Parmesan cheese for serving (optional)
- Lemon wedges for serving (optional)

Cooking Instructions:
1. Preheat the oven to 400°F (200°C). Line a baking sheet with parchment paper or aluminum foil.

2. In a large mixing bowl, toss Brussels sprouts with olive oil, minced garlic, salt, and pepper until evenly coated.

3. Spread the Brussels sprouts in a single layer on the prepared baking sheet.

4. Roast in the preheated oven for 20-25 minutes, or until the Brussels sprouts are tender and caramelized, stirring halfway through cooking.

5. Remove from the oven and transfer the roasted Brussels sprouts to a serving dish.

6. If desired, sprinkle with grated Parmesan cheese and serve hot with lemon wedges on the side.

Cook Tips:

- For extra flavor, you can add balsamic vinegar or honey to the olive oil mixture before tossing with the Brussels sprouts.

- To ensure even cooking, make sure the Brussels sprouts are cut into similar-sized pieces.

Nutritional Value:

- Brussels sprouts are a nutritious vegetable that is rich in fiber, vitamins C and K, and antioxidants, making them an excellent side dish for any meal. Roasting Brussels sprouts enhances their natural sweetness and caramelizes the edges, resulting in a delicious and flavorful side dish that is sure to please your taste buds while providing essential nutrition to support your health and well-being during your cancer journey.

Steamed Broccoli with Lemon

Ingredients:
- 1 pound broccoli florets
- 2 tablespoons water
- 1 tablespoon olive oil
- 1 teaspoon lemon zest
- 1 tablespoon fresh lemon juice
- Salt and pepper to taste

Cooking Instructions:
1. Place broccoli florets in a microwave-safe dish with 2 tablespoons of water.
2. Cover the dish with a microwave-safe lid or plate and microwave on high for 3-4 minutes, or until the broccoli is tender-crisp.

3. Carefully remove the dish from the microwave and drain any excess water.

4. Drizzle olive oil over the steamed broccoli and sprinkle with lemon zest and fresh lemon juice.

5. Season with salt and pepper to taste, and toss gently to coat.

6. Serve the steamed broccoli hot as a nutritious and flavorful side dish.

Cook Tips:

- To steam broccoli on the stovetop, place broccoli florets in a steamer basket over boiling water and cover with a lid. Steam for 5-7 minutes, or until tender-crisp.

- Customize the dish by adding minced garlic or red pepper flakes for extra flavor.

Nutritional Value:

- Broccoli is a nutrient-dense vegetable that is rich in vitamins, minerals, and antioxidants, making it an excellent choice for a healthy side dish. Steaming broccoli helps retain its vibrant green color and crisp texture while preserving its nutritional value. Drizzled with olive oil and fresh lemon juice, this simple yet delicious side dish is sure to brighten up any meal while providing essential nutrition to support your health and well-being during your cancer journey.

These dinner recipes from "The Great Cancer Diet Cookbook" are designed to provide nourishment, flavor, and enjoyment during your cancer journey. By incorporating a variety of nutrient-rich ingredients into your meals and focusing on wholesome, balanced options, you can support your health and well-being while satisfying your taste buds. Whether you're looking for a balanced main course, a plant-based protein option, or a healthy side dish, these recipes offer something for everyone. Enjoy these delicious and nutritious dinner options

Snacks and Appetizers for Cancer Patients

Snacks and appetizers are important components of a balanced diet, providing nourishment and energy between meals. These recipes from "The Great Cancer Diet Cookbook" are designed to be both delicious and nutritious, offering a variety of options to support your health and well-being during your cancer journey.

Nutrient-Dense Snacks

Nutrient-dense snacks are packed with vitamins, minerals, and antioxidants to support your health and provide sustained energy throughout the day. These recipes feature wholesome ingredients that are easy to prepare and perfect for satisfying hunger between meals.

Almond and Date Energy Balls

Ingredients:
- 1 cup almonds
- 1 cup pitted dates
- 1 tablespoon almond butter
- 1 tablespoon honey or maple syrup
- 1 teaspoon vanilla extract
- Pinch of sea salt
- Optional add-ins: shredded coconut, cocoa powder, chopped nuts, dried fruit

Cooking Instructions:
1. In a food processor, pulse almonds until finely ground.
2. Add pitted dates, almond butter, honey or maple syrup, vanilla extract, and sea salt to the food processor.
3. Process until the mixture comes together and forms a sticky dough.
4. If desired, add optional add-ins such as shredded coconut, cocoa powder, chopped nuts, or dried fruit, and pulse until combined.
5. Using your hands, roll the mixture into small balls and place them on a parchment-lined baking sheet.

6. Refrigerate for at least 30 minutes to firm up.
7. Serve the almond and date energy balls chilled as a nutritious and satisfying snack.

Cook Tips:
- To make it easier to blend, soak the dates in warm water for 10-15 minutes before using.
- Customize the energy balls by rolling them in cocoa powder, shredded coconut, or chopped nuts for added flavor and texture.

Nutritional Value:
- Almonds are a rich source of healthy fats, protein, and fiber, while dates provide natural sweetness and energy-boosting carbohydrates. Combined with almond butter, honey or maple syrup, and vanilla extract, these energy balls offer a delicious and nutritious snack option that is perfect for satisfying hunger and providing sustained energy between meals.

Veggie Chips

Ingredients:
- Assorted vegetables (such as sweet potatoes, beets, carrots, zucchini, and kale)
- Olive oil
- Salt and pepper
- Optional seasonings: garlic powder, onion powder, paprika, cumin, chili powder

Cooking Instructions:
1. Preheat the oven to 375°F (190°C). Line a baking sheet with parchment paper or aluminum foil.
2. Wash and dry the assorted vegetables. Peel and slice the vegetables thinly using a mandoline slicer or sharp knife.
3. In a large mixing bowl, toss the sliced vegetables with olive oil until evenly coated.
4. Arrange the vegetable slices in a single layer on the prepared baking sheet.
5. Season with salt, pepper, and optional seasonings according to your taste preferences.
6. Bake in the preheated oven for 10-15 minutes, or until the vegetable chips are

golden brown and crispy, flipping halfway through cooking.

7. Remove from the oven and let cool slightly before serving.

Cook Tips:

- Keep an eye on the vegetable chips while baking to prevent them from burning. Thinner slices will cook more quickly than thicker ones.

- Experiment with different vegetables and seasonings to create your own unique flavor combinations.

Nutritional Value:

- Veggie chips offer a healthier alternative to traditional potato chips, providing vitamins, minerals, and antioxidants from a variety of colorful vegetables. Baked instead of fried, these crispy chips are lower in fat and calories, making them a nutritious and guilt-free snack option that is perfect for munching on between meals.

Healthy Dips and Spreads

Healthy dips and spreads add flavor and nutrition to your snacks and appetizers, making them more satisfying and enjoyable to eat. These recipes feature wholesome ingredients that are easy to prepare and perfect for dipping veggies, crackers, or whole grain bread.

Classic Hummus

Ingredients:
- 1 can (15 ounces) chickpeas, drained and rinsed
- 2 tablespoons tahini
- 2 tablespoons olive oil
- 2 cloves garlic, minced
- 2 tablespoons fresh lemon juice
- 1/4 teaspoon ground cumin
- Salt and pepper to taste
- Water, as needed

Cooking Instructions:

1. In a food processor, combine chickpeas, tahini, olive oil, minced garlic, fresh lemon juice, ground cumin, salt, and pepper.

2. Process until smooth and creamy, scraping down the sides of the bowl as needed.

3. If the hummus is too thick, add water, 1 tablespoon at a time, until desired consistency is reached.

4. Taste and adjust seasoning as needed.

5. Transfer the hummus to a serving bowl and drizzle with additional olive oil, if desired.

6. Serve the classic hummus with vegetable sticks, pita bread, or crackers for dipping.

Cook Tips:

- For extra flavor, you can add roasted red peppers, sun-dried tomatoes, or fresh herbs such as parsley or cilantro to the hummus.

- Store leftover hummus in an airtight container in the refrigerator for up to one week.

Nutritional Value:

- Hummus is a nutritious and versatile dip made from chickpeas, tahini, olive oil, and garlic, providing protein, fiber, healthy fats, and essential nutrients. Paired with vegetable sticks or whole grain crackers, this classic hummus recipe offers a delicious and satisfying snack option that is perfect for dipping and sharing with family and friends.

Avocado and White Bean Dip

Ingredients:
- 1 ripe avocado, peeled and pitted
- 1 can (15 ounces) white beans, drained and rinsed
- 2 cloves garlic, minced
- 2 tablespoons fresh lemon juice
- 2 tablespoons olive oil
- 1/4 teaspoon ground cumin
- Salt and pepper to taste
- Optional garnishes: chopped fresh cilantro, diced tomatoes, sliced green onions

Cooking Instructions:
1. In a food processor, combine ripe avocado, white beans, minced garlic, fresh lemon juice, olive oil, ground cumin, salt, and pepper.

2. Process until smooth and creamy, scraping down the sides of the bowl as needed.

3. Taste and adjust seasoning as needed.

4. Transfer the avocado and white bean dip to a serving bowl and garnish with optional toppings such as chopped fresh cilantro, diced tomatoes, or sliced green onions.

5. Serve the dip with vegetable sticks, whole grain crackers,or pita bread for dipping.

Cook Tips:

- For added creaminess, you can add a dollop of Greek yogurt or sour cream to the dip.

- Customize the dip by adding other ingredients such as roasted garlic, jalapeno peppers, or fresh herbs like parsley or basil.

Nutritional Value:

- Avocado and white bean dip combines the creamy texture of avocado with the protein and fiber-rich white beans, providing a nutritious and flavorful dip that is perfect for snacking. Packed with vitamins, minerals, and healthy fats, this dip offers a satisfying option for dipping vegetables, crackers, or pita bread, while supporting your health and well-being during your cancer journey.

Simple Appetizers

Simple appetizers are perfect for entertaining or enjoying as a light snack before a meal. These recipes feature easy-to-make dishes that are full of flavor and nutrition, making them ideal for any occasion.

Stuffed Mushrooms

Ingredients:
- 12 large mushrooms, stems removed and reserved
- 1 tablespoon olive oil
- 2 cloves garlic, minced
- 1/4 cup onion, finely chopped
- 1/4 cup breadcrumbs
- 1/4 cup grated Parmesan cheese
- 2 tablespoons fresh parsley, chopped
- Salt and pepper to taste

Cooking Instructions:

1. Preheat the oven to 375°F (190°C). Lightly grease a baking sheet with olive oil or cooking spray.

2. Finely chop the reserved mushroom stems.

3. In a skillet, heat olive oil over medium heat. Add minced garlic and chopped onion, and sauté until softened, about 5 minutes.

4. Add chopped mushroom stems to the skillet and cook for an additional 3-4 minutes, or until tender.

5. Remove the skillet from heat and stir in breadcrumbs, grated Parmesan cheese, chopped parsley, salt, and pepper.

6. Spoon the filling into the mushroom caps, pressing down gently to pack the filling.

7. Place the stuffed mushrooms on the prepared baking sheet.

8. Bake in the preheated oven for 15-20 minutes, or until the mushrooms are tender and the filling is golden brown.

9. Remove from the oven and let cool slightly before serving.

Cook Tips:
- For a vegetarian option, omit the Parmesan cheese or use a plant-based alternative.
- Experiment with different herbs and spices to customize the flavor of the stuffing.

Nutritional Value:
- Stuffed mushrooms are a tasty and nutritious appetizer that is perfect for any occasion. Mushrooms are a good source of vitamins, minerals, and antioxidants, while the filling adds flavor and texture to the dish. With a crispy breadcrumb topping and savory Parmesan cheese, these stuffed mushrooms are sure to be a hit with your family and friends while providing essential nutrition to support your health and well-being during your cancer journey.

Caprese Skewers

Ingredients:
- Cherry or grape tomatoes
- Fresh mozzarella cheese, cut into bite-sized pieces
- Fresh basil leaves

- Balsamic glaze or reduction
- Wooden skewers

Assembly Instructions:
1. Thread one cherry tomato, one piece of fresh mozzarella cheese, and one fresh basil leaf onto each wooden skewer, repeating until all ingredients are used.
2. Arrange the caprese skewers on a serving platter.
3. Drizzle balsamic glaze or reduction over the skewers just before serving.
4. Serve the caprese skewers immediately as a simple and elegant appetizer.

Cook Tips:
- Choose ripe cherry or grape tomatoes and fresh mozzarella cheese for the best flavor and texture.
- If you don't have wooden skewers, you can serve the caprese ingredients on toothpicks or cocktail picks for bite-sized appetizers.

Nutritional Value:
- Caprese skewers are a classic Italian appetizer that combines the vibrant flavors of

ripe tomatoes, creamy mozzarella cheese, and aromatic basil. Drizzled with balsamic glaze or reduction, these skewers offer a burst of flavor and freshness that is perfect for any occasion. With their simple yet elegant presentation, caprese skewers are sure to impress your guests while providing essential nutrition to support your health and well-being during your cancer journey.

These snacks and appetizers from "The Great Cancer Diet Cookbook" are designed to provide nourishment, flavor, and enjoyment during your cancer journey. By incorporating a variety of nutrient-rich ingredients into your snacks and appetizers and focusing on wholesome, balanced options, you can support your health and well-being while satisfying your taste buds. Whether you're looking for a nutrient-dense snack, a healthy dip or spread, or a simple appetizer, these recipes offer something for everyone. Enjoy these delicious and nutritious snack and appetizer options as part of your daily routine, and remember to listen to your body and eat according to your individual needs and preferences.

Desserts for Cancer Patients

Indulging in desserts can still be a part of a healthy diet for cancer patients. These recipes from "The Great Cancer Diet Cookbook" are designed to satisfy your sweet tooth while providing essential nutrients and supporting your overall well-being during your cancer journey.

Guilt-Free Treats

Guilt-free treats are delicious desserts made with wholesome ingredients to satisfy your cravings without compromising your health. These recipes feature nutrient-rich ingredients that are perfect for indulging in a guilt-free dessert.

Dark Chocolate Avocado Mousse

Ingredients:
- 2 ripe avocados, peeled and pitted
- 1/4 cup cocoa powder
- 1/4 cup maple syrup or honey

- 1 teaspoon vanilla extract
- Pinch of sea salt
- Optional toppings: sliced strawberries, shaved dark chocolate, chopped nuts

Cooking Instructions:
1. In a food processor or blender, combine ripe avocados, cocoa powder, maple syrup or honey, vanilla extract, and sea salt.
2. Process until smooth and creamy, scraping down the sides of the bowl as needed.
3. Taste and adjust sweetness as needed by adding more maple syrup or honey.
4. Transfer the avocado mousse to serving bowls or glasses.
5. Refrigerate for at least 30 minutes to chill before serving.
6. Serve the dark chocolate avocado mousse chilled, topped with sliced strawberries, shaved dark chocolate, or chopped nuts if desired.

Cook Tips:
- Make sure the avocados are ripe for a smoother texture and sweeter flavor.

- For a creamier consistency, you can add a splash of coconut milk or almond milk to the mousse.

Nutritional Value:
- Dark chocolate avocado mousse is a rich and creamy dessert that is packed with healthy fats, fiber, and antioxidants. Avocados provide a velvety texture and essential nutrients, while cocoa powder adds a rich chocolate flavor without the added sugar. Topped with fresh fruit or nuts, this guilt-free treat is sure to satisfy your sweet cravings while providing essential nutrition to support your health and well-being during your cancer journey.

Baked Apples with Cinnamon

Ingredients:
- 4 apples, cored
- 2 tablespoons maple syrup or honey
- 1 teaspoon ground cinnamon
- Optional toppings: chopped nuts, dried fruit, Greek yogurt, or coconut whipped cream

Cooking Instructions:

1. Preheat the oven to 375°F (190°C). Lightly grease a baking dish with olive oil or cooking spray.
2. Place cored apples in the prepared baking dish.
3. In a small bowl, whisk together maple syrup or honey and ground cinnamon.
4. Drizzle the cinnamon mixture over the apples, making sure to coat them evenly.
5. Bake in the preheated oven for 30-40 minutes, or until the apples are tender and caramelized.
6. Remove from the oven and let cool slightly before serving.
7. Serve the baked apples warm, topped with optional toppings such as chopped nuts, dried fruit, Greek yogurt, or coconut whipped cream.

Cook Tips:

- Choose firm apples such as Granny Smith or Honeycrisp for the best results.
- Customize the flavor of the baked apples by adding a sprinkle of nutmeg or cloves along with the cinnamon.

Nutritional Value:
- Baked apples with cinnamon are a simple yet satisfying dessert that is perfect for any occasion. Apples are a good source of fiber, vitamins, and antioxidants, while cinnamon adds warm and aromatic flavor without the added sugar. Whether enjoyed on their own or topped with your favorite toppings, these baked apples are sure to please your taste buds while providing essential nutrition to support your health and well-being during your cancer journey.

Fruit-Based Desserts

Fruit-based desserts are naturally sweet and refreshing options that are perfect for satisfying your sweet tooth while providing essential vitamins and minerals. These recipes feature a variety of fruits paired with simple ingredients to create delicious and nutritious desserts.

Berry Parfait

Ingredients:
- 1 cup Greek yogurt or dairy-free yogurt alternative
- 1 cup mixed berries (such as strawberries, blueberries, raspberries)
- 1/4 cup granola or toasted oats
- 1 tablespoon honey or maple syrup
- Optional toppings: shredded coconut, chopped nuts, fresh mint leaves

Assembly Instructions:
1. In a serving glass or bowl, layer Greek yogurt, mixed berries, and granola or toasted oats.
2. Drizzle honey or maple syrup over the top of the parfait.
3. Repeat layers until the glass or bowl is filled.
4. Garnish with optional toppings such as shredded coconut, chopped nuts, or fresh mint leaves.
5. Serve the berry parfait immediately as a refreshing and nutritious dessert.

Cook Tips:
- Use your favorite combination of berries for the parfait, or choose seasonal fruits for the best flavor.
- For a vegan option, use dairy-free yogurt and omit the honey or maple syrup.

Nutritional Value:
- Berry parfait is a light and refreshing dessert that is packed with vitamins, minerals, and antioxidants from fresh fruit and Greek yogurt. Berries are low in calories and high in fiber, making them an excellent choice for satisfying your sweet cravings without the added sugar. Layered with creamy yogurt and crunchy granola, this parfait offers a satisfying texture and delicious flavor that is perfect for enjoying any time of day while providing essential nutrition to support your health and well-being during your cancer journey.

Grilled Pineapple with Honey

Ingredients:
- 1 pineapple, peeled and sliced into rings

- 2 tablespoons honey
- Optional toppings: Greek yogurt, coconut whipped cream, chopped nuts, fresh mint leaves

Cooking Instructions:
1. Preheat the grill or grill pan over medium-high heat.
2. Place pineapple rings on the preheated grill and cook for 2-3 minutes per side, or until grill marks appear and the pineapple is caramelized.
3. Remove the grilled pineapple from the grill and transfer to a serving platter.
4. Drizzle honey over the grilled pineapple.
5. Serve the grilled pineapple warm, topped with optional toppings such as Greek yogurt, coconut whipped cream, chopped nuts, or fresh mint leaves.

Cook Tips:
- Choose ripe pineapple for the best flavor and sweetness.
- If you don't have a grill, you can also broil the pineapple in the oven or cook it in a grill pan on the stovetop.

Nutritional Value:

- Grilled pineapple with honey is a simple yet delicious dessert that is perfect for summer cookouts or backyard barbecues. Pineapple is rich in vitamin C, manganese, and bromelain, an enzyme that may have anti-inflammatory properties. Grilling caramelizes the natural sugars in the pineapple, enhancing its sweetness and flavor. Drizzled with honey and topped with optional toppings, this dessert offers a satisfyingly sweet and tangy treat that is sure to please your taste buds while providing essential nutrition to support your health and well-being during your cancer journey.

Healthy Baking

Healthy baking allows you to enjoy your favorite treats without the guilt by using wholesome ingredients and simple cooking techniques. These recipes feature nutritious ingredients that are perfect for baking delicious and satisfying desserts.

Almond Flour Cookies

Ingredients:
- 2 cups almond flour
- 1/4 cup coconut oil, melted
- 1/4 cup maple syrup or honey
- 1 teaspoonvanilla extract
- 1/4 teaspoon baking soda
- Pinch of salt
- Optional add-ins: dark chocolate chips, chopped nuts, dried fruit

Cooking Instructions:
1. Preheat the oven to 350°F (175°C). Line a baking sheet with parchment paper.
2. In a mixing bowl, combine almond flour, melted coconut oil, maple syrup or honey, vanilla extract, baking soda, and salt.
3. Mix until a dough forms. If the dough is too dry, add a splash of almond milk to moisten.
4. Fold in optional add-ins such as dark chocolate chips, chopped nuts, or dried fruit.
5. Scoop tablespoon-sized portions of dough and roll them into balls. Place them on the prepared baking sheet.

6. Flatten each cookie slightly with the palm of your hand.

7. Bake in the preheated oven for 10-12 minutes, or until the edges are golden brown.

8. Remove from the oven and let the cookies cool on the baking sheet for 5 minutes before transferring them to a wire rack to cool completely.

Cook Tips:

- Almond flour can vary in texture, so adjust the amount of liquid (coconut oil or almond milk) as needed to achieve the right consistency for the cookie dough.
- For a chewier texture, underbake the cookies slightly.

Nutritional Value:

- Almond flour cookies are a delicious and nutritious treat that is perfect for satisfying your sweet cravings while providing essential nutrients. Almond flour is rich in healthy fats, protein, and fiber, making it a healthier alternative to traditional wheat flour. Sweetened with natural sweeteners like maple syrup or honey and flavored with vanilla extract, these cookies offer a deliciously nutty flavor and soft texture that is sure to please your taste buds while providing essential nutrition to support your health and well-being during your cancer journey.

Carrot and Walnut Muffins

Ingredients:
- 1 1/2 cups almond flour
- 1/2 cup coconut flour
- 1 teaspoon baking soda
- 1 teaspoon ground cinnamon
- 1/4 teaspoon ground nutmeg
- Pinch of salt
- 3 eggs, beaten
- 1/4 cup coconut oil, melted
- 1/4 cup maple syrup or honey
- 1 teaspoon vanilla extract
- 1 cup grated carrots
- 1/2 cup chopped walnuts
- Optional add-ins: raisins, shredded coconut, grated apple

Cooking Instructions:

1. Preheat the oven to 350°F (175°C). Line a muffin tin with paper liners or grease with coconut oil.

2. In a large mixing bowl, whisk together almond flour, coconut flour, baking soda, ground cinnamon, ground nutmeg, and salt.

3. In a separate bowl, combine beaten eggs, melted coconut oil, maple syrup or honey, and vanilla extract.

4. Pour the wet ingredients into the dry ingredients and stir until just combined.

5. Fold in grated carrots, chopped walnuts, and optional add-ins such as raisins, shredded coconut, or grated apple.

6. Divide the muffin batter evenly among the prepared muffin cups, filling each about 3/4 full.

7. Bake in the preheated oven for 20-25 minutes, or until the muffins are golden brown and a toothpick inserted into the center comes out clean.

8. Remove from the oven and let the muffins cool in the tin for 5 minutes before transferring them to a wire rack to cool completely.

Cook Tips:
- Be careful not to overmix the batter, as this can result in dense muffins.
- For a sweeter flavor, you can add more maple syrup or honey, or increase the amount of dried fruit in the muffins.

Nutritional Value:
- Carrot and walnut muffins are a wholesome and satisfying treat that is perfect for breakfast or as a snack. Made with almond flour and coconut flour, these muffins are gluten-free and grain-free, making them suitable for those with dietary restrictions. Loaded with grated carrots, chopped walnuts, and warming spices like cinnamon and nutmeg, these muffins offer a deliciously moist texture and sweet flavor that is sure to please your taste buds while providing essential nutrition to support your health and well-being during your cancer journey.

These dessert recipes from "The Great Cancer Diet Cookbook" prove that indulging in sweets can still be part of a healthy diet for cancer patients. By using wholesome ingredients and simple cooking techniques, you can create delicious and satisfying desserts that nourish your body and support your overall well-being during your cancer journey. Whether you're craving something rich and chocolatey or something light and fruity, these dessert options offer something for everyone to enjoy while providing essential nutrition to support your health and well-being.

Healing Drinks for Cancer Patients

Staying hydrated is essential for cancer patients, and incorporating healing drinks into your daily routine can provide a flavorful and nutritious way to support your health and well-being. These recipes from "The Great Cancer Diet Cookbook" feature a variety of healing teas, refreshing smoothies, and hydrating beverages to nourish your body and promote healing during your cancer journey.

Healing Teas and Infusions

Healing teas and infusions are soothing beverages that can provide comfort and relief during your cancer treatment. These recipes feature ingredients known for their anti-inflammatory and antioxidant properties, making them ideal for supporting your health and well-being.

Turmeric Ginger Tea

Ingredients:
- 1 inch piece of fresh ginger, peeled and thinly sliced
- 1 teaspoon ground turmeric
- 4 cups water
- 1 tablespoon honey (optional)
- Juice of 1/2 lemon (optional)

Cooking Instructions:
1. In a small saucepan, combine sliced ginger, ground turmeric, and water.
2. Bring the mixture to a boil over medium-high heat.
3. Reduce the heat to low and simmer for 10-15 minutes, allowing the flavors to infuse.
4. Remove from heat and strain the tea into mugs.
5. Stir in honey and lemon juice if desired.
6. Serve the turmeric ginger tea hot and enjoy its soothing and healing properties.

Cook Tips:
- Adjust the amount of honey and lemon juice according to your taste preferences.

- For added flavor, you can add a cinnamon stick or a few cloves to the tea while simmering.

Nutritional Value:
- Turmeric ginger tea is a warm and comforting beverage that is known for its anti-inflammatory and immune-boosting properties. Ginger and turmeric contain bioactive compounds such as gingerol and curcumin, which have been studied for their potential health benefits, including reducing inflammation and supporting digestion. Enjoying a cup of turmeric ginger tea can provide soothing relief and promote healing during your cancer journey.

Green Tea with Lemon

Ingredients:
- 2 green tea bags
- 4 cups water
- Juice of 1 lemon
- Honey or stevia to taste (optional)

Brewing Instructions:
1. Bring 4 cups of water to a boil in a kettle or saucepan.
2. Place green tea bags in a teapot or heatproof pitcher.
3. Pour the boiling water over the tea bags and let steep for 3-5 minutes.
4. Remove the tea bags and discard.
5. Stir in lemon juice and sweeten with honey or stevia if desired.
6. Pour the green tea into mugs and serve hot, or let it cool and refrigerate for iced tea.

Cook Tips:
- Green tea can become bitter if steeped for too long, so avoid overbrewing.
- For a refreshing twist, add a few sprigs of fresh mint to the tea while steeping.

Nutritional Value:
- Green tea with lemon is a light and refreshing beverage that is rich in antioxidants and nutrients. Green tea contains catechins, a type of antioxidant that may help protect cells from damage and reduce inflammation. Adding lemon juice to green tea

not only enhances its flavor but also provides vitamin C, which supports immune function and promotes healing. Enjoying a cup of green tea with lemon can provide a refreshing boost of hydration and essential nutrients during your cancer journey.

Refreshing Smoothies and Juices

Refreshing smoothies and juices are an easy and delicious way to incorporate fruits and vegetables into your diet while staying hydrated. These recipes feature a variety of nutrient-rich ingredients that are perfect for supporting your health and well-being during your cancer journey.

Cucumber Mint Juice

Ingredients:
- 1 cucumber, peeled and chopped
- Handful of fresh mint leaves
- 1/2 lemon, peeled and seeded
- 1 cup water or coconut water
- Ice cubes (optional)

Blending Instructions:
1. Place chopped cucumber, fresh mint leaves, peeled lemon, and water or coconut water in a blender.
2. Blend on high speed until smooth and creamy.
3. If desired, add ice cubes and blend again until well combined.
4. Pour the cucumber mint juice into glasses and serve immediately.

Cook Tips:
- For a sweeter flavor, you can add a small amount of honey or stevia to the juice.
- Customize the juice by adding other ingredients such as ginger, celery, or spinach.

Nutritional Value:
- Cucumber mint juice is a refreshing and hydrating beverage that is perfect for staying cool and replenishing fluids during your cancer journey. Cucumbers are low in calories and high in water content, making them a hydrating choice, while fresh mint adds a burst of flavor and may help soothe digestion. Adding lemon provides a tangy kick of vitamin

C, which supports immune function and promotes healing. Enjoying a glass of cucumber mint juice can provide essential hydration and nutrients to support your health and well-being.

Beet and Carrot Juice

Ingredients:
- 2 medium beets, peeled and chopped
- 4 carrots, peeled and chopped
- 1 apple, cored and chopped
- 1 inch piece of fresh ginger, peeled
- 1 lemon, peeled and seeded
- 1 cup water or coconut water
- Ice cubes (optional)

Blending Instructions:
1. Place chopped beets, carrots, apple, ginger, and lemon in a blender.
2. Add water or coconut water to the blender.
3. Blend on high speed until smooth and well combined.
4. If desired, add ice cubes and blend again until smooth.

5. Pour the beet and carrot juice into glasses and serve immediately.

Cook Tips:
- To prevent staining, wear gloves when handling beets or wash your hands immediately after.
- Adjust the sweetness of the juice by adding more or fewer apples.

Nutritional Value:
- Beet and carrot juice is a vibrant and nutrient-rich beverage that is packed with vitamins, minerals, and antioxidants. Beets are rich in betalains, compounds that have been studied for their potential anti-inflammatory and antioxidant properties, while carrots provide beta-carotene, which is converted into vitamin A in the body and supports immune function. Adding apple, ginger, and lemon enhances the flavor of the juice and provides additional nutrients and immune-boosting properties. Enjoying a glass of beet and carrot juice can provide essential nutrients and

hydration to support your health and well-being during your cancer journey.

Hydrating Beverages

Hydrating beverages are essential for maintaining optimal hydration and supporting overall health and well-being during your cancer journey. These recipes feature hydrating ingredients that are perfect for quenching your thirst and replenishing fluids.

Coconut Water and Berry Cooler

Ingredients:
- 1 cup coconut water
- 1/2 cup mixed berries (such as strawberries, blueberries, raspberries)
- Juice of 1/2 lime
- 1 tablespoon honey or maple syrup (optional)
- Ice cubes (optional)

Assembly Instructions:
1. In a blender, combine coconut water, mixed berries, lime juice, and honey or maple syrup if desired.
2. Blend on high speed until smooth and well combined.
3. If desired, add ice cubes to the blender and blend again until chilled.
4. Pour the coconut water and berry cooler into glasses and serveimmediately.

Cook Tips:
- Choose ripe and sweet berries for the best flavor.
- If you prefer a sweeter taste, you can add more honey or maple syrup.

Nutritional Value:
- Coconut water and berry cooler is a refreshing and hydrating beverage that is perfect for staying cool and replenishing fluids during your cancer journey. Coconut water is naturally rich in electrolytes such as potassium and magnesium, which help maintain fluid balance and support hydration. Mixed berries add a burst of flavor and provide

vitamins, minerals, and antioxidants that support immune function and promote healing. Adding lime juice enhances the flavor of the cooler and provides a refreshing citrus twist. Enjoying a glass of coconut water and berry cooler can provide essential hydration and nutrients to support your health and well-being.

Lemon and Mint Infused Water

Ingredients:
- 1 lemon, thinly sliced
- Handful of fresh mint leaves
- 4 cups water
- Ice cubes (optional)

Assembly Instructions:
1. In a pitcher, combine lemon slices and fresh mint leaves.
2. Fill the pitcher with water.
3. Refrigerate for at least 1 hour to allow the flavors to infuse.
4. If desired, add ice cubes to the pitcher before serving to chill the infused water further.

5. Serve the lemon and mint infused water in glasses over ice.

Cook Tips:
- For a stronger flavor, muddle the mint leaves slightly before adding them to the pitcher.
- You can customize the infused water by adding other ingredients such as cucumber slices, ginger, or berries.

Nutritional Value:
- Lemon and mint infused water is a refreshing and hydrating beverage that is perfect for quenching your thirst and supporting your health and well-being during your cancer journey. Lemon provides a tangy flavor and vitamin C, which supports immune function and promotes healing. Fresh mint adds a cooling and refreshing element to the infused water and may help soothe digestion. Enjoying a glass of lemon and mint infused water can provide essential hydration and nutrients while offering a flavorful and refreshing alternative to plain water.

Incorporating healing drinks into your daily routine can provide a flavorful and nutritious way to support your health and well-being during your cancer journey. Whether you prefer soothing teas, refreshing smoothies, or hydrating beverages, these recipes from "The Great Cancer Diet Cookbook" offer a variety of options to suit your taste preferences and dietary needs. By choosing ingredients rich in antioxidants, vitamins, and minerals, you can nourish your body and promote healing while enjoying delicious and satisfying beverages. Cheers to your health and well-being!

PART III: SPECIAL DIETS AND CONSIDERATIONS

Special Diets for Cancer Patients

Cancer treatment can often come with a range of side effects that can affect appetite, taste, and the ability to eat certain foods. In "The Great Cancer Diet Cookbook," we provide recipes tailored to manage these side effects and cater to specific dietary restrictions. From combating nausea to accommodating dietary preferences, these recipes are designed to support cancer patients in maintaining a nutritious diet during their treatment journey.

Managing Side Effects Through Diet

Certain side effects of cancer treatment, such as nausea, appetite loss, mouth sores, and swallowing difficulties, can impact a patient's ability to eat and enjoy meals. These recipes are carefully crafted to alleviate these symptoms and provide nourishment when it's needed most.

Recipes for Nausea and Appetite Loss

Dealing with nausea and appetite loss can be challenging during cancer treatment, but incorporating the right foods into your diet can help alleviate these symptoms and provide much-needed nourishment. These recipes from "The Great Cancer Diet Cookbook" are carefully crafted to soothe the stomach and stimulate the appetite, making mealtime more enjoyable and satisfying.

Ginger Chicken Soup

Ingredients:
- 2 boneless, skinless chicken breasts
- 4 cups chicken broth
- 1 tablespoon fresh ginger, grated
- 2 carrots, chopped
- 1 celery stalk, chopped
- 1 cup cooked rice or quinoa
- Salt and pepper to taste
- Fresh parsley for garnish (optional)

Cooking Instructions:

1. In a large pot, bring the chicken broth to a simmer over medium heat.

2. Add the chicken breasts, grated ginger, carrots, and celery to the pot.

3. Cover and simmer for 20-25 minutes, or until the chicken is cooked through.

4. Remove the chicken breasts from the pot and shred them using two forks.

5. Return the shredded chicken to the pot and add cooked rice or quinoa.

6. Season with salt and pepper to taste.

7. Simmer for an additional 5-10 minutes to allow the flavors to meld.

8. Serve the ginger chicken soup hot, garnished with fresh parsley if desired.

Cook Tips:

- Ginger is known for its anti-nausea properties and can help soothe an upset stomach. Adding fresh ginger to the soup enhances its flavor and makes it more digestible for patients experiencing nausea.

- If appetite loss is an issue, try serving the soup in smaller portions throughout the day to make it more manageable.

Nutritional Value:
- Ginger chicken soup is a comforting and nourishing dish that is gentle on the stomach and easy to digest. Chicken provides lean protein, which is essential for maintaining muscle mass and strength during cancer treatment. Carrots and celery add fiber and essential vitamins and minerals, while ginger offers anti-inflammatory and digestive benefits. Enjoying a bowl of ginger chicken soup can provide warmth and comfort while helping to alleviate nausea and stimulate the appetite.

Creamy Butternut Squash Soup

Ingredients:
- 1 medium butternut squash, peeled, seeded, and diced
- 1 onion, diced
- 2 cloves garlic, minced
- 4 cups vegetable broth
- 1/2 cup coconut milk
- 1 tablespoon olive oil
- Salt and pepper to taste

- Fresh thyme for garnish (optional)

Cooking Instructions:
1. In a large pot, heat olive oil over medium heat.
2. Add diced onion and minced garlic to the pot and sauté until softened, about 5 minutes.
3. Add diced butternut squash and vegetable broth to the pot.
4. Bring to a boil, then reduce heat and simmer for 20-25 minutes, or until the squash is fork-tender.
5. Use an immersion blender to puree the soup until smooth and creamy.
6. Stir in coconut milk and season with salt and pepper to taste.
7. Simmer for an additional 5 minutes to heat through.
8. Serve the creamy butternut squash soup hot, garnished with fresh thyme if desired.

Cook Tips:
- Pureed soups are ideal for patients experiencing mouth sores or swallowing difficulties, as they require minimal chewing and are easier to swallow.

– For added protein and texture, you can stir in cooked quinoa or lentils before serving.

Nutritional Value:
– Creamy butternut squash soup is a soothing and nourishing dish that is perfect for patients experiencing mouth sores or swallowing difficulties. Butternut squash is rich in vitamins A and C, which support immune function and promote healing. Coconut milk adds creaminess and healthy fats, while onions and garlic provide flavor and anti-inflammatory benefits. Enjoying a bowl of creamy butternut squash soup can provide essential nutrients and comfort while supporting your health and well-being during your cancer journey.

Recipes for Mouth Sores and Swallowing Difficulties

Mouth sores and swallowing difficulties can make eating a challenging and uncomfortable experience for cancer patients. However, incorporating soft, soothing, and easy-to-swallow foods into your diet can help alleviate these symptoms and ensure you're getting the nourishment your body needs. These recipes from "The Great Cancer Diet Cookbook" are designed specifically to provide relief for mouth sores and swallowing difficulties while still being delicious and nutritious.

Creamy Mashed Sweet Potatoes

Ingredients:
- 2 large sweet potatoes, peeled and diced
- 2 tablespoons unsalted butter or olive oil
- 1/4 cup milk or non-dairy milk
- Salt and pepper to taste
- Fresh parsley or chives for garnish (optional)

Cooking Instructions:
1. Place the diced sweet potatoes in a large pot and cover with water.
2. Bring the water to a boil, then reduce heat to medium-low and simmer for 15-20 minutes, or until the sweet potatoes are fork-tender.

3. Drain the sweet potatoes and return them to the pot.
4. Add butter or olive oil, milk, salt, and pepper to the pot.
5. Use a potato masher or fork to mash the sweet potatoes until smooth and creamy.
6. If the mashed sweet potatoes are too thick, you can add more milk or a splash of broth to reach your desired consistency.
7. Serve the creamy mashed sweet potatoes hot, garnished with fresh parsley or chives if desired.

Cook Tips:
- For patients experiencing mouth sores, avoid adding any spices or seasonings that may irritate the mouth. Keep the mashed sweet potatoes simple with just butter, milk, salt, and pepper.
- If swallowing difficulties are an issue, you can puree the mashed sweet potatoes in a blender or food processor until smooth.

Nutritional Value:
- Creamy mashed sweet potatoes are a soft and comforting dish that is gentle on the

mouth and easy to swallow. Sweet potatoes are rich in vitamins A and C, which support immune function and promote healing. Adding butter or olive oil provides healthy fats, while milk adds creaminess and a boost of calcium. Enjoying a serving of creamy mashed sweet potatoes can provide essential nutrients and comfort during your cancer journey.

Silky Butternut Squash Soup

Ingredients:
- 1 medium butternut squash, peeled, seeded, and diced
- 1 onion, diced
- 2 cloves garlic, minced
- 4 cups vegetable broth
- 1/2 cup coconut milk
- 1 tablespoon olive oil
- Salt and pepper to taste
- Fresh thyme for garnish (optional)

Cooking Instructions:
1. In a large pot, heat olive oil over medium heat.

2. Add diced onion and minced garlic to the pot and sauté until softened, about 5 minutes.
3. Add diced butternut squash and vegetable broth to the pot.
4. Bring to a boil, then reduce heat and simmer for 20-25 minutes, or until the squash is fork-tender.
5. Use an immersion blender to puree the soup until smooth and creamy.
6. Stir in coconut milk and season with salt and pepper to taste.
7. Simmer for an additional 5 minutes to heat through.
8. Serve the silky butternut squash soup hot, garnished with fresh thyme if desired.

Cook Tips:
- Pureed soups are ideal for patients experiencing mouth sores or swallowing difficulties, as they require minimal chewing and are easier to swallow.
- For added protein and texture, you can stir in cooked quinoa or lentils before serving.

Nutritional Value:
- Silky butternut squash soup is a soothing and nourishing dish that is perfect for patients experiencing mouth sores or swallowing difficulties. Butternut squash is rich in vitamins A and C, which support immune function and promote healing. Coconut milk adds creaminess and healthy fats, while onions and garlic provide flavor and anti-inflammatory benefits. Enjoying a bowl of silky butternut squash soup can provide essential nutrients and comfort while supporting your health and well-being during your cancer journey.

Diet Modifications for Specific Cancers

Different types of cancer may require specific dietary modifications to support treatment and overall health. These recipes are tailored to the nutritional needs and preferences of patients with breast cancer and prostate cancer.

Recipes for Breast Cancer Patients

Breast cancer patients often undergo rigorous treatments that can affect their appetite, energy levels, and overall well-being. It's crucial for them to maintain a nutritious diet to support their recovery and boost their immune system. These recipes from "The Great Cancer Diet Cookbook" are specially curated to provide breast cancer patients with delicious and nourishing meals that are packed with essential nutrients to aid in their healing journey.

Roasted Salmon with Lemon and Dill

Ingredients:
- 4 salmon fillets, skin-on
- 2 tablespoons olive oil
- 2 cloves garlic, minced
- Zest of 1 lemon
- Juice of 1 lemon
- 2 tablespoons fresh dill, chopped
- Salt and pepper to taste

Cooking Instructions:
1. Preheat your oven to 400°F (200°C).
2. Place the salmon fillets skin-side down on a baking sheet lined with parchment paper.
3. In a small bowl, whisk together the olive oil, minced garlic, lemon zest, lemon juice, and chopped dill.
4. Brush the lemon-dill mixture over the salmon fillets, coating them evenly.
5. Season the salmon with salt and pepper to taste.
6. Roast in the preheated oven for 12-15 minutes, or until the salmon is cooked through and flakes easily with a fork.
7. Remove from the oven and let the salmon rest for a few minutes before serving.
8. Serve the roasted salmon hot, garnished with additional fresh dill and lemon slices if desired.

Cook Tips:
- Choose wild-caught salmon for its higher omega-3 fatty acid content, which has been shown to have anti-inflammatory properties and may help reduce the risk of cancer recurrence.

- Be careful not to overcook the salmon to prevent it from becoming dry. Check for doneness by gently inserting a fork into the thickest part of the fillet – it should flake easily.

Nutritional Value:
- Salmon is an excellent source of protein and omega-3 fatty acids, which are essential for muscle repair and reducing inflammation in the body. The addition of lemon and dill not only enhances the flavor of the dish but also provides a boost of vitamin C and antioxidants. Enjoying a serving of roasted salmon with lemon and dill can provide breast cancer patients with a delicious and nutritious meal that supports their recovery and overall health.

Quinoa and Kale Salad with Lemon-Tahini Dressing

Ingredients:
- 1 cup quinoa, rinsed
- 2 cups water or vegetable broth
- 4 cups kale, stems removed and chopped

- 1 cucumber, diced
- 1 bell pepper, diced
- 1/4 cup red onion, thinly sliced
- 1/4 cup fresh parsley, chopped

Lemon-Tahini Dressing:
- 1/4 cup tahini
- Juice of 1 lemon
- 2 tablespoons olive oil
- 1 tablespoon maple syrup or honey
- 1 clove garlic, minced
- Salt and pepper to taste

Cooking Instructions:
1. In a medium saucepan, combine the quinoa and water or vegetable broth. Bring to a boil, then reduce heat to low, cover, and simmer for 15-20 minutes, or until the quinoa is cooked and the liquid is absorbed. Remove from heat and let it cool slightly.
2. In a large mixing bowl, combine the cooked quinoa, chopped kale, diced cucumber, diced bell pepper, sliced red onion, and chopped parsley.
3. In a small bowl, whisk together the tahini, lemon juice, olive oil, maple syrup or honey,

minced garlic, salt, and pepper until smooth and creamy.

4. Pour the lemon-tahini dressing over the quinoa and kale salad, tossing until well coated.

5. Serve the salad immediately, or refrigerate for at least 30 minutes to allow the flavors to meld before serving.

Cook Tips:

- Massaging the kale with a bit of olive oil and lemon juice before adding it to the salad can help soften its texture and reduce bitterness.

- Feel free to customize the salad by adding your favorite vegetables, nuts, seeds, or protein sources such as grilled chicken or chickpeas.

Nutritional Value:

- Quinoa is a gluten-free whole grain that is rich in protein, fiber, and essential vitamins and minerals, making it an excellent choice for breast cancer patients. Kale is packed with antioxidants, vitamins, and minerals, including vitamin C, vitamin K, and calcium, which support immune function and bone health. The lemon-tahini dressing adds creaminess and tanginess to the salad while providing healthy fats and flavor. Enjoying a serving of quinoa and kale salad with lemon-tahini dressing can provide breast cancer patients with a nutritious and satisfying meal that supports their recovery and well-being.

These recipes are specifically tailored to the nutritional needs of breast cancer patients, providing them with delicious and nourishing options to support their healing journey. Incorporating these dishes into their diet can help them maintain their strength, energy levels, and overall health as they undergo treatment and recovery.

Recipes for Prostate Cancer Patients

Prostate cancer patients often face unique dietary challenges, and maintaining a healthy diet is essential for supporting their treatment and recovery. These recipes from "The Great Cancer Diet Cookbook" are carefully crafted to provide prostate cancer patients with delicious and nourishing meals that promote overall health and well-being. From antioxidant-rich ingredients to prostate-friendly foods, these recipes are designed to support prostate health and enhance the body's natural defenses against cancer.

Grilled Salmon with Garlic and Herbs

Ingredients:
- 4 salmon fillets, skin-on
- 2 tablespoons olive oil
- 2 cloves garlic, minced
- 1 tablespoon fresh parsley, chopped
- 1 tablespoon fresh dill, chopped
- 1 tablespoon fresh thyme, chopped
- Salt and pepper to taste
- Lemon wedges for serving

Cooking Instructions:
1. Preheat your grill to medium-high heat.
2. In a small bowl, combine the olive oil, minced garlic, chopped parsley, dill, and thyme.

3. Brush the herb mixture over the salmon fillets, coating them evenly.

4. Season the salmon with salt and pepper to taste.

5. Place the salmon fillets skin-side down on the preheated grill.

6. Grill for 4-5 minutes per side, or until the salmon is cooked through and flakes easily with a fork.

7. Remove from the grill and let the salmon rest for a few minutes before serving.

8. Serve the grilled salmon hot, with lemon wedges on the side for squeezing over the fish.

Cook Tips:

- Choose wild-caught salmon for its higher omega-3 fatty acid content, which has been shown to have anti-inflammatory properties and may help reduce the risk of prostate cancer progression.

- Avoid charring the salmon, as charred or burnt foods may contain carcinogens. Aim for a golden-brown crust on the outside while keeping the inside tender and moist.

Nutritional Value:
- Grilled salmon is a lean source of protein and heart-healthy omega-3 fatty acids, which are beneficial for prostate health. Garlic and herbs not only enhance the flavor of the dish but also provide antioxidant and anti-inflammatory properties. Enjoying a serving of grilled salmon with garlic and herbs can provide prostate cancer patients with essential nutrients and support their overall well-being.

Quinoa Salad with Roasted Vegetables and Balsamic Vinaigrette

Ingredients:
- 1 cup quinoa, rinsed
- 2 cups water or vegetable broth
- 2 cups mixed vegetables (such as bell peppers, zucchini, cherry tomatoes, and red onion), chopped
- 2 tablespoons olive oil
- Salt and pepper to taste

Balsamic Vinaigrette:
- 3 tablespoons balsamic vinegar

- 2 tablespoons olive oil
- 1 teaspoon Dijon mustard
- 1 clove garlic, minced
- Salt and pepper to taste

Cooking Instructions:
1. Preheat your oven to 400°F (200°C).
2. In a medium saucepan, combine the quinoa and water or vegetable broth. Bring to a boil, then reduce heat to low, cover, and simmer for 15-20 minutes, or until the quinoa is cooked and the liquid is absorbed. Remove from heat and let it cool slightly.
3. Meanwhile, spread the chopped vegetables on a baking sheet lined with parchment paper.
4. Drizzle olive oil over the vegetables and season with salt and pepper to taste.
5. Roast in the preheated oven for 20-25 minutes, or until the vegetables are tender and lightly caramelized.
6. In a small bowl, whisk together the balsamic vinegar, olive oil, Dijon mustard, minced garlic, salt, and pepper to make the vinaigrette.

7. In a large mixing bowl, combine the cooked quinoa, roasted vegetables, and balsamic vinaigrette. Toss until well coated.
8. Serve the quinoa salad warm or chilled, garnished with fresh herbs if desired.

Cook Tips:
- Roasting the vegetables brings out their natural sweetness and enhances their flavor. Feel free to use your favorite vegetables or whatever is in season.
- Make a big batch of quinoa salad and store it in the refrigerator for easy meal prep throughout the week. It makes a satisfying and nutritious meal on its own or as a side dish.

Nutritional Value:
- Quinoa is a gluten-free whole grain that is rich in protein, fiber, and essential nutrients, making it an excellent choice for prostate cancer patients. Mixed vegetables provide a variety of vitamins, minerals, and antioxidants that support overall health and immune function. The balsamic vinaigrette adds a tangy and savory flavor to the salad

while providing heart-healthy fats and antioxidants. Enjoying a serving of quinoa salad with roasted vegetables and balsamic vinaigrette can provide prostate cancer patients with a delicious and nutritious meal that supports their recovery and well-being

Recipes for Common Dietary Restrictions: Gluten-Free Options

Maintaining a gluten-free diet is essential for individuals with celiac disease or gluten intolerance. However, many people choose to follow a gluten-free lifestyle for various health reasons, including cancer patients seeking to reduce inflammation and digestive discomfort. These gluten-free recipes from "The Great Cancer Diet Cookbook" are not only safe for those with gluten restrictions but are also delicious and nutritious options for all cancer patients to enjoy.

1. Quinoa-Stuffed Bell Peppers

Ingredients:
- 4 large bell peppers, any color

- 1 cup quinoa, rinsed
- 2 cups vegetable broth
- 1 tablespoon olive oil
- 1 onion, diced
- 2 cloves garlic, minced
- 1 zucchini, diced
- 1 cup cherry tomatoes, halved
- 1/2 cup corn kernels (fresh, frozen, or canned)
- 1/4 cup fresh parsley, chopped
- 1/4 cup fresh basil, chopped
- Salt and pepper to taste
- 1/2 cup shredded cheese (optional, for topping)

Cooking Instructions:
1. Preheat your oven to 375°F (190°C).
2. Cut the tops off the bell peppers and remove the seeds and membranes. Place the peppers upright in a baking dish.
3. In a medium saucepan, combine the quinoa and vegetable broth. Bring to a boil, then reduce heat to low, cover, and simmer for 15–20 minutes, or until the quinoa is cooked and the liquid is absorbed. Remove from heat and set aside.

4. In a large skillet, heat olive oil over medium heat. Add diced onion and minced garlic, and sauté until softened, about 5 minutes.

5. Add diced zucchini to the skillet and cook for an additional 3-4 minutes, until tender.

6. Stir in cherry tomatoes, corn kernels, cooked quinoa, chopped parsley, and chopped basil. Season with salt and pepper to taste.

7. Spoon the quinoa mixture into the hollowed-out bell peppers, pressing down gently to pack the filling.

8. If using shredded cheese, sprinkle it over the stuffed peppers.

9. Cover the baking dish with foil and bake in the preheated oven for 25-30 minutes, or until the peppers are tender.

10. Remove the foil and bake for an additional 5-10 minutes, until the cheese is melted and bubbly (if using).

11. Serve the quinoa-stuffed bell peppers hot, garnished with additional fresh herbs if desired.

Cook Tips:
- Choose bell peppers that are firm and evenly colored for the best results.

- Feel free to customize the filling with your favorite vegetables or protein sources. Mushrooms, spinach, black beans, or cooked ground turkey are all excellent additions.

Nutritional Value:
- Quinoa is a gluten-free whole grain that is rich in protein, fiber, and essential nutrients, making it an ideal option for those following a gluten-free diet. Bell peppers are packed with vitamin C, vitamin A, and antioxidants, which support immune function and overall health. This dish provides a balanced combination of carbohydrates, protein, and fiber, making it a satisfying and nutritious meal for cancer patients. Enjoying a serving of quinoa-stuffed bell peppers can provide essential nutrients while satisfying your appetite and taste buds.

2. **Gluten-Free Chicken and Vegetable Stir-Fry**

Ingredients:
- 2 boneless, skinless chicken breasts, thinly sliced

- 2 tablespoons gluten-free soy sauce or tamari
- 1 tablespoon rice vinegar
- 1 tablespoon honey or maple syrup
- 1 tablespoon olive oil
- 2 cloves garlic, minced
- 1 tablespoon fresh ginger, grated
- 1 red bell pepper, sliced
- 1 yellow bell pepper, sliced
- 1 cup broccoli florets
- 1 carrot, julienned
- 1/2 cup snow peas
- Cooked rice or quinoa, for serving

Cooking Instructions:
1. In a small bowl, whisk together the gluten-free soy sauce or tamari, rice vinegar, and honey or maple syrup. Set aside.
2. Heat olive oil in a large skillet or wok over medium-high heat. Add minced garlic and grated ginger, and cook for 1-2 minutes until fragrant.
3. Add sliced chicken breasts to the skillet and cook until browned and cooked through, about 5-7 minutes.

4. Remove the cooked chicken from the skillet and set aside.

5. In the same skillet, add sliced bell peppers, broccoli florets, julienned carrot, and snow peas. Cook for 5-6 minutes, stirring frequently, until the vegetables are tender-crisp.

6. Return the cooked chicken to the skillet and pour the soy sauce mixture over the chicken and vegetables. Stir well to combine and coat everything in the sauce.

7. Cook for an additional 2-3 minutes, until the sauce has thickened slightly.

8. Serve the gluten-free chicken and vegetable stir-fry hot, over cooked rice or quinoa.

Cook Tips:

- For a gluten-free option, use tamari instead of soy sauce, as it is made without wheat and is suitable for those with gluten sensitivities.

- Feel free to add or substitute your favorite vegetables in this stir-fry. Bell peppers, broccoli, carrots, and snow peas are classic choices, but you can also include mushrooms, snap peas, or baby corn.

Nutritional Value:
- This gluten-free chicken and vegetable stir-fry is a balanced and nutritious meal that provides protein, fiber, and an array of vitamins and minerals. Chicken is a lean source of protein, while vegetables like bell peppers, broccoli, and carrots are rich in vitamin C, vitamin A, and antioxidants. Serving the stir-fry over cooked rice or quinoa adds complex carbohydrates to keep you feeling satisfied and energized. Enjoying a serving of this gluten-free stir-fry can provide cancer patients with essential nutrients while satisfying their cravings for a flavorful and comforting meal.

3. **Gluten-Free Quinoa Salad with Lemon-Herb Dressing**

Ingredients:
- 1 cup quinoa, rinsed
- 2 cups water or vegetable broth
- 1 cucumber, diced
- 1 pint cherry tomatoes, halved
- 1/4 cup red onion, thinly sliced
- 1/4 cup fresh parsley, chopped

- 1/4 cup fresh mint, chopped
- 1/4 cup crumbled feta cheese (optional)
- Salt and pepper to taste

Lemon-Herb Dressing:
- 1/4 cup olive oil
- Juice of 1 lemon
- 1 tablespoon honey or maple syrup
- 1 clove garlic, minced
- 1 teaspoon Dijon mustard
- 1 tablespoon fresh parsley, chopped
- 1 tablespoon fresh mint, chopped
- Salt and pepper to taste

Cooking Instructions:
1. In a medium saucepan, combine the quinoa and vegetable broth. Bring to a boil, then reduce heat to low, cover, and simmer for 15-20 minutes, or until the quinoa is cooked and the liquid is absorbed. Remove from heat and let it cool slightly.
2. In a large mixing bowl, combine the cooked quinoa, diced cucumber, halved cherry tomatoes, thinly sliced red onion, chopped parsley, and chopped mint.

3. In a small bowl, whisk together the olive oil, lemon juice, honey or maple syrup, minced garlic, Dijon mustard, chopped parsley, chopped mint, salt, and pepper to make the lemon-herb dressing.

4. Pour the dressing over the quinoa salad and toss until well coated.

5. If using, sprinkle crumbled feta cheese over the salad and gently toss to combine.

6. Taste and adjust seasoning with salt and pepper if needed.

7. Serve the gluten-free quinoa salad with lemon-herb dressing chilled or at room temperature.

Cook Tips:

- Rinse the quinoa thoroughly before cooking to remove any bitter taste.

- Make sure to let the quinoa cool slightly before adding the vegetables and dressing to prevent them from wilting.

- Customize the salad by adding your favorite ingredients such as olives, avocado, or grilled chicken for extra protein.

Nutritional Value:
- Quinoa is a gluten-free whole grain that is high in protein, fiber, and essential nutrients, making it a nutritious base for this salad. Cucumbers and cherry tomatoes add freshness and hydration, while red onion provides a pop of flavor and crunch. Fresh herbs like parsley and mint not only enhance the taste but also provide antioxidants and anti-inflammatory properties. The lemon-herb dressing adds brightness and tanginess to the salad, making it a refreshing and satisfying dish for cancer patients following a gluten-free diet. Enjoying a serving of this quinoa salad can provide essential nutrients while supporting overall health and well-being.

4. Gluten-Free Zucchini Noodles with Pesto Sauce

Ingredients:
- 4 medium zucchinis
- 1 tablespoon olive oil
- 1/4 cup pine nuts, toasted
- 2 cups fresh basil leaves

- 1/4 cup grated Parmesan cheese (optional)
- 2 cloves garlic
- Juice of 1 lemon
- Salt and pepper to taste

Cooking Instructions:
1. Use a spiralizer to spiralize the zucchinis into noodles. Alternatively, you can use a julienne peeler to create thin strips.
2. Heat olive oil in a large skillet over medium heat. Add the zucchini noodles and sauté for 2-3 minutes, or until just tender.
3. In a food processor or blender, combine the toasted pine nuts, fresh basil leaves, grated Parmesan cheese (if using), garlic cloves, lemon juice, salt, and pepper. Pulse until smooth and well combined.
4. Toss the cooked zucchini noodles with the pesto sauce until evenly coated.
5. Serve the gluten-free zucchini noodles with pesto sauce immediately, garnished with additional pine nuts and grated Parmesan cheese if desired.

Cook Tips:
- Be careful not to overcook the zucchini noodles, as they can become mushy. They should be tender but still have a slight crunch.
- Feel free to customize the pesto sauce by adding other ingredients such as spinach, kale, or roasted red peppers for extra flavor and nutrients.
- Store any leftover pesto sauce in an airtight container in the refrigerator for up to one week or freeze it for longer storage.

Nutritional Value:
- Zucchini noodles are a low-carb, gluten-free alternative to traditional pasta, making them perfect for cancer patients following a gluten-free diet. They are rich in vitamins, minerals, and antioxidants, which support immune function and overall health. Pesto sauce made with fresh basil provides a burst of flavor and is packed with vitamins A, C, and K, as well as essential nutrients like iron and calcium. Enjoying a serving of gluten-free zucchini noodles with pesto sauce can provide cancer patients with a satisfying

and nutritious meal that supports their dietary needs and taste preferences.

5. Gluten-Free Banana-Oat Muffins

Ingredients:
- 2 cups gluten-free rolled oats
- 1 teaspoon baking powder
- 1/2 teaspoon baking soda
- 1/2 teaspoon ground cinnamon
- 1/4 teaspoon salt
- 2 ripe bananas, mashed
- 2 large eggs
- 1/4 cup maple syrup or honey
- 1/4 cup unsweetened applesauce
- 1/4 cup unsweetened almond milk
- 1 teaspoon vanilla extract
- Optional add-ins: chopped nuts, dried fruit, chocolate chips

Cooking Instructions:
1. Preheat your oven to 350°F (175°C). Line a muffin tin with paper liners or lightly grease with cooking spray.

2. In a blender or food processor, pulse the gluten-free rolled oats until they form a fine flour-like consistency.

3. In a large mixing bowl, whisk together the oat flour, baking powder, baking soda, ground cinnamon, and salt.

4. In a separate bowl, mash the ripe bananas with a fork until smooth. Add the eggs, maple syrup or honey, unsweetened applesauce, unsweetened almond milk, and vanilla extract. Mix until well combined.

5. Pour the wet ingredients into the dry ingredients and stir until just combined. Be careful not to overmix.

6. If using any optional add-ins, gently fold them into the muffin batter.

7. Divide the batter evenly among the prepared muffin cups, filling each about three-quarters full.

8. Bake in the preheated oven for 18-20 minutes, or until the muffins are golden brown and a toothpick inserted into the center comes out clean.

9. Remove from the oven and let the muffins cool in the tin for 5 minutes before

transferring them to a wire rack to cool completely.

Cook Tips:
- Make sure to use certified gluten-free oats to ensure the muffins are entirely gluten-free.
- Feel free to customize the muffins by adding your favorite mix-ins such as chopped nuts, dried fruit, or chocolate chips.
- Store any leftover muffins in an airtight container at room temperature for up to three days or freeze them for longer storage.

Nutritional Value:
- These gluten-free banana-oat muffins are made with wholesome ingredients like oats, bananas, and eggs, making them a nutritious option for cancer patients following a gluten-free diet. Oats are high in fiber and contain beta-glucan, a type of soluble fiber that has been shown to support heart health and regulate blood sugar levels. Bananas provide natural sweetness and are a good source of potassium, vitamin C, and vitamin B6. Enjoying a serving of these gluten-free banana-oat muffins can provide cancer

patients with a tasty and satisfying treat that meets their dietary needs and supports their overall well-being.

These five gluten-free recipes offer flavorful and nutritious options for cancer patients looking to maintain a healthy diet while following a gluten-free lifestyle. Whether you're cooking for yourself or a loved one, these recipes are sure to please the palate while nourishing the body.

Dairy-Free Recipes for Cancer Patients

Maintaining a dairy-free diet can be essential for cancer patients with lactose intolerance or dairy allergies. Additionally, some individuals choose to avoid dairy to reduce inflammation or digestive discomfort. These dairy-free recipes from "The Great Cancer Diet Cookbook" are not only safe for those with dairy restrictions but are also delicious and nutritious options for all cancer patients to enjoy.

1. Dairy-Free Creamy Tomato Basil Soup

Ingredients:
- 2 tablespoons olive oil
- 1 onion, chopped
- 2 cloves garlic, minced
- 2 carrots, chopped
- 2 celery stalks, chopped
- 1 can (28 oz) diced tomatoes
- 2 cups vegetable broth
- 1 can (14 oz) coconut milk (full-fat)
- 1/4 cup fresh basil leaves, chopped
- Salt and pepper to taste

Cooking Instructions:
1. Heat olive oil in a large pot over medium heat. Add chopped onion and garlic, and sauté until softened, about 5 minutes.
2. Add chopped carrots and celery to the pot, and cook for an additional 5 minutes, until slightly tender.
3. Pour in the diced tomatoes (with their juices) and vegetable broth. Bring to a boil, then reduce heat and simmer for 15-20 minutes, until the vegetables are fully cooked.

4. Using an immersion blender, puree the soup until smooth and creamy.

5. Stir in the coconut milk and chopped basil. Season with salt and pepper to taste.

6. Cook for an additional 5 minutes, allowing the flavors to meld together.

7. Serve the dairy-free creamy tomato basil soup hot, garnished with additional fresh basil leaves if desired.

Cook Tips:

- Use full-fat coconut milk for a creamy texture and rich flavor.

- If you don't have an immersion blender, carefully transfer the soup to a blender in batches and blend until smooth. Be sure to allow the soup to cool slightly before blending to prevent splattering.

Nutritional Value:

- This dairy-free creamy tomato basil soup is rich in antioxidants, vitamins, and minerals. Tomatoes are a great source of lycopene, a powerful antioxidant that may help protect against certain types of cancer. Coconut milk adds creaminess and healthy fats, while fresh basil provides a burst of flavor and additional antioxidants. Enjoying a serving of this soup can provide cancer patients with essential nutrients while soothing the palate and nourishing the body.

2. Dairy-Free Vegetable Stir-Fry with Tofu

Ingredients:
- 1 block (14 oz) extra-firm tofu, pressed and cubed
- 2 tablespoons soy sauce or tamari
- 1 tablespoon sesame oil
- 2 tablespoons olive oil
- 2 cloves garlic, minced
- 1 tablespoon fresh ginger, grated
- 2 cups broccoli florets
- 1 red bell pepper, sliced
- 1 yellow bell pepper, sliced
- 1 cup snap peas
- Cooked rice or quinoa, for serving

Cooking Instructions:
1. In a large mixing bowl, toss the cubed tofu with soy sauce (or tamari) and sesame oil until

evenly coated. Let marinate for 15-20 minutes.

2. Heat olive oil in a large skillet or wok over medium-high heat. Add minced garlic and grated ginger, and cook for 1-2 minutes until fragrant.

3. Add marinated tofu to the skillet and cook until browned and crispy on all sides, about 5-7 minutes. Remove the tofu from the skillet and set aside.

4. In the same skillet, add broccoli florets, sliced bell peppers, and snap peas. Cook for 5-6 minutes, stirring frequently, until the vegetables are tender-crisp.

5. Return the cooked tofu to the skillet and toss with the vegetables until evenly combined.

6. Serve the dairy-free vegetable stir-fry hot, over cooked rice or quinoa.

Cook Tips:
- Pressing the tofu before cooking helps remove excess moisture, allowing it to crisp up nicely when cooked.

- Customize the stir-fry by adding your favorite vegetables such as mushrooms, carrots, or baby corn.

Nutritional Value:
- This dairy-free vegetable stir-fry with tofu is packed with protein, fiber, and an array of vitamins and minerals. Tofu is a plant-based source of protein that provides essential amino acids necessary for tissue repair and immune function. Mixed vegetables like broccoli, bell peppers, and snap peas add color, texture, and a variety of nutrients to the dish. Serving the stir-fry over cooked rice or quinoa adds complex carbohydrates to keep you feeling satisfied and energized. Enjoying a serving of this dairy-free stir-fry can provide cancer patients with essential nutrients while satisfying their cravings for a flavorful and nutritious meal.

3. Dairy-Free Avocado Pasta

Ingredients:
- 8 oz gluten-free pasta (such as brown rice or quinoa pasta)

- 2 ripe avocados, peeled and pitted
- 1/4 cup fresh basil leaves
- 2 cloves garlic, minced
- Juice of 1 lemon
- 2 tablespoons olive oil
- Salt and pepper to taste
- Optional toppings: cherry tomatoes, pine nuts, chopped fresh basil

Cooking Instructions:
1. Cook the gluten-free pasta according to the package instructions until al dente. Drain and set aside.
2. In a food processor or blender, combine the ripe avocados, fresh basil leaves, minced garlic, lemon juice, olive oil, salt, and pepper. Blend until smooth and creamy.
3. Toss the cooked pasta with the dairy-free avocado sauce until evenly coated.
4. Serve the dairy-free avocado pasta hot, garnished with cherry tomatoes, pine nuts, and chopped fresh basil if desired.

Cook Tips:
- Reserve some pasta cooking water to thin out the sauce if needed.

- Feel free to add additional ingredients to the pasta such as grilled chicken, shrimp, or roasted vegetables for extra protein and flavor.

Nutritional Value:
- This dairy-free avocado pasta is a creamy and satisfying dish that is rich in heart-healthy fats, vitamins, and minerals. Avocados are a great source of monounsaturated fats, which may help lower cholesterol levels and reduce inflammation. Fresh basil adds a burst of flavor and is rich in antioxidants and essential oils. Serving the pasta over gluten-free noodles provides complex carbohydrates and fiber, which can help stabilize blood sugar levels and promote digestive health. Enjoying a serving of this dairy-free avocado pasta can provide cancer patients with essential nutrients while supporting their overall well-being and dietary preferences.

4. Dairy-Free Lentil Soup

Ingredients:
- 1 cup dried green or brown lentils, rinsed and drained
- 1 onion, chopped
- 2 carrots, chopped
- 2 celery stalks, chopped
- 2 cloves garlic, minced
- 6 cups vegetable broth
- 1 can (14 oz) diced tomatoes
- 1 teaspoon ground cumin
- 1/2 teaspoon ground turmeric
- 1/2 teaspoon smoked paprika
- Salt and pepper to taste
- Fresh parsley, chopped (for garnish)

Cooking Instructions:
1. In a large pot, heat olive oil over medium heat. Add chopped onion, carrots, and celery, and cook until softened, about 5-7 minutes.
2. Add minced garlic to the pot and cook for an additional minute, until fragrant.
3. Add dried lentils, vegetable broth, diced tomatoes (with their juices), ground cumin,

ground turmeric, smoked paprika, salt, and pepper to the pot. Stir to combine.

4. Bring the soup to a boil, then reduce heat to low and simmer for 25-30 minutes, or until the lentils are tender.

5. Taste and adjust seasoning with salt and pepper if needed.

6. Serve the dairy-free lentil soup hot, garnished with fresh chopped parsley.

Cook Tips:

- For added flavor, you can sauté the vegetables in a combination of olive oil and vegetable broth instead of just olive oil.

- Feel free to customize the soup by adding other vegetables such as potatoes, sweet potatoes, or spinach.

Nutritional Value:

- This dairy-free lentil soup is a hearty and nutritious dish that is rich in plant-based protein, fiber, and essential nutrients. Lentils are a great source of protein and fiber, which can help support digestion, stabilize blood sugar levels, and promote satiety. Carrots and celery provide vitamins, minerals, and antioxidants, while diced tomatoes add acidity and depth of flavor to the soup. Spices like cumin, turmeric, and smoked paprika add warmth and complexity to the dish. Enjoying a serving of this dairy-free lentil soup can provide cancer patients with essential nutrients while satisfying their hunger and nourishing their bodies.

5. Dairy-Free Banana Bread

Ingredients:
- 2 ripe bananas, mashed
- 1/4 cup coconut oil, melted
- 1/4 cup maple syrup or honey
- 2 eggs
- 1 teaspoon vanilla extract
- 1 1/2 cups gluten-free flour (such as almond flour or oat flour)
- 1 teaspoon baking powder
- 1/2 teaspoon baking soda
- 1/2 teaspoon ground cinnamon
- Pinch of salt
- Optional add-ins: chopped nuts, chocolate chips, dried fruit

Cooking Instructions:

1. Preheat your oven to 350°F (175°C). Grease a loaf pan with coconut oil or line with parchment paper.

2. In a large mixing bowl, combine mashed bananas, melted coconut oil, maple syrup or honey, eggs, and vanilla extract. Mix until well combined.

3. In a separate bowl, whisk together gluten-free flour, baking powder, baking soda, ground cinnamon, and salt.

4. Gradually add the dry ingredients to the wet ingredients, stirring until just combined. Be careful not to overmix.

5. If using any optional add-ins, gently fold them into the banana bread batter.

6. Pour the batter into the prepared loaf pan and smooth the top with a spatula.

7. Bake in the preheated oven for 50-60 minutes, or until a toothpick inserted into the center comes out clean.

8. Remove from the oven and let the banana bread cool in the pan for 10 minutes before transferring it to a wire rack to cool completely.

Cook Tips:
- Make sure your bananas are ripe for the best flavor and sweetness.
- If using almond flour, be aware that the texture of the banana bread may be denser compared to using oat flour.
- Store any leftover banana bread in an airtight container at room temperature for up to three days or freeze it for longer storage.

Nutritional Value:
- This dairy-free banana bread is a wholesome and delicious treat that is perfect for breakfast or as a snack. Ripe bananas provide natural sweetness and moisture to the bread, while coconut oil adds richness and healthy fats. Gluten-free flour ensures that the bread is suitable for those with gluten sensitivities or allergies. Enjoying a slice of this dairy-free banana bread can provide cancer patients with a comforting and satisfying indulgence while adhering to their dietary needs and preferences.

These five dairy-free recipes offer flavorful and nourishing options for cancer patients seeking delicious alternatives to dairy-based dishes. Whether you're looking for soups, entrees, or baked goods, these recipes are sure to please the palate and support your health and well-being.

Recipes for Immune Support

Cancer patients often experience weakened immune systems due to treatment and the disease itself. Incorporating immune-boosting ingredients into their diet can help strengthen their immune response and promote overall wellness. These recipes from "The Great Cancer Diet Cookbook" feature ingredients known for their immune-boosting properties and are designed to nourish the body and support immune health.

Immune-Boosting Ingredients

1. Garlic, Ginger, and Turmeric:
   - Garlic contains compounds like allicin, which have antimicrobial and immune-boosting properties.
   - Ginger has anti-inflammatory and antioxidant properties that can help support immune function.

- Turmeric contains curcumin, a potent antioxidant with anti-inflammatory and immune-modulating effects.

2. Leafy Greens and Berries:

- Leafy greens like spinach, kale, and Swiss chard are rich in vitamins, minerals, and antioxidants that support immune health.

- Berries such as strawberries, blueberries, and raspberries are packed with vitamin C, antioxidants, and flavonoids that help strengthen the immune system.

Simple Recipes to Strengthen Immunity

1. Garlic and Ginger Chicken Soup

Ingredients:
- 1 tablespoon olive oil
- 1 onion, diced
- 3 cloves garlic, minced
- 1-inch piece of ginger, grated
- 2 carrots, sliced
- 2 celery stalks, sliced
- 6 cups chicken or vegetable broth
- 2 cups cooked shredded chicken

- 1 cup spinach leaves
- Salt and pepper to taste
- Fresh parsley, chopped (for garnish)

Cooking Instructions:
1. In a large pot, heat olive oil over medium heat. Add diced onion, minced garlic, and grated ginger. Sauté until fragrant, about 2-3 minutes.
2. Add sliced carrots and celery to the pot, and cook for another 5 minutes until slightly softened.
3. Pour in chicken or vegetable broth and bring to a simmer. Let it cook for 10-15 minutes until the vegetables are tender.
4. Add cooked shredded chicken to the pot and simmer for an additional 5 minutes until heated through.
5. Stir in spinach leaves and cook until wilted, about 1-2 minutes.
6. Season with salt and pepper to taste.
7. Ladle the garlic and ginger chicken soup into bowls and garnish with chopped fresh parsley before serving.

Cook Tips:
- For an extra immune boost, add additional immune-boosting ingredients like turmeric or lemon juice to the soup.
- Make a large batch of this soup and store it in individual portions in the freezer for easy reheating on busy days.

Nutritional Value:
- This garlic and ginger chicken soup is a comforting and nourishing dish that is rich in immune-boosting ingredients. Garlic and ginger provide antimicrobial and anti-inflammatory benefits, while chicken broth provides essential nutrients and hydration. Adding vegetables like carrots, celery, and spinach adds vitamins, minerals, and antioxidants to support overall health. Enjoying a serving of this soup can help strengthen the immune system and provide cancer patients with the nutrients they need to thrive.

2. **Turmeric and Black Pepper Smoothie**

Ingredients:
- 1 cup unsweetened almond milk or coconut milk
- 1 ripe banana
- 1/2 cup frozen pineapple chunks
- 1/2 teaspoon ground turmeric
- 1/4 teaspoon ground cinnamon
- Pinch of black pepper
- 1 tablespoon chia seeds or flaxseeds (optional)
- Honey or maple syrup to taste (optional)

Cooking Instructions:
1. In a blender, combine almond milk, ripe banana, frozen pineapple chunks, ground turmeric, ground cinnamon, black pepper, and chia seeds or flaxseeds if using.
2. Blend on high until smooth and creamy.
3. Taste and adjust sweetness with honey or maple syrup if desired.
4. Pour the turmeric and black pepper smoothie into glasses and serve immediately.

Cook Tips:
- Black pepper helps enhance the absorption of curcumin, the active compound in turmeric, so be sure to include a pinch in your smoothie.
- Customize your smoothie by adding other immune-boosting ingredients like spinach, kale, or berries.

Nutritional Value:
- This turmeric and black pepper smoothie is a refreshing and nutritious beverage that is packed with immune-boosting ingredients. Turmeric contains curcumin, a potent antioxidant with anti-inflammatory and immune-modulating effects. Black pepper helps improve the bioavailability of curcumin, making it more readily absorbed by the body. Pineapple adds natural sweetness and vitamin C, while banana provides potassium and fiber. Enjoying a glass of this smoothie can provide cancer patients with a delicious way to support their immune system and overall well-being.

These simple recipes featuring immune-boosting ingredients like garlic, ginger, turmeric, leafy greens, and berries are designed to strengthen the immune system and support the health and well-being of cancer patients. Incorporating these recipes into your meal plan can help provide the essential nutrients needed to promote immune health and enhance overall vitality.

Recipes for Weight Management

Maintaining a healthy weight is crucial for cancer patients as it supports overall well-being and can aid in managing treatment side effects. Whether you're looking to gain weight or maintain a healthy weight, these recipes from "The Great Cancer Diet Cookbook" are designed to provide nourishment and support your weight management goals.

Healthy Weight Gain Recipes

1. Protein-Rich Smoothies

Ingredients:
- 1 cup full-fat coconut milk or almond milk
- 1 ripe banana
- 1/2 cup Greek yogurt or dairy-free yogurt alternative
- 1 scoop protein powder (whey protein, pea protein, or hemp protein)
- 1 tablespoon almond butter or peanut butter
- 1 tablespoon chia seeds or flaxseeds

- Optional add-ins: spinach, kale, berries, avocado

Cooking Instructions:
1. In a blender, combine coconut milk or almond milk, ripe banana, Greek yogurt or dairy-free yogurt alternative, protein powder, almond butter or peanut butter, and chia seeds or flaxseeds.
2. Add any optional add-ins like spinach, kale, berries, or avocado for extra nutrition.
3. Blend on high until smooth and creamy.
4. Taste and adjust sweetness or thickness by adding more banana or liquid if needed.
5. Pour the protein-rich smoothie into glasses and serve immediately.

Cook Tips:
- Customize your smoothie based on your taste preferences and nutritional needs. Experiment with different fruits, vegetables, and protein powders to find your favorite combination.
- To increase the calorie content of your smoothie, add additional nut butter, avocado, or a drizzle of honey or maple syrup.

Nutritional Value:
- Protein-rich smoothies are an excellent option for cancer patients looking to gain weight as they provide a concentrated source of calories, protein, and essential nutrients. Coconut milk or almond milk adds creaminess and healthy fats, while Greek yogurt or dairy-free yogurt alternative contributes protein and probiotics for gut health. Adding protein powder boosts the protein content of the smoothie, which is essential for tissue repair and muscle maintenance. Enjoying a protein-rich smoothie as a meal or snack can help support weight gain and provide cancer patients with the nourishment they need to thrive.

2. Calorie-Dense Snacks

Ingredients:
- Nuts and seeds (almonds, walnuts, cashews, pumpkin seeds, sunflower seeds)
- Nut butter (almond butter, peanut butter, cashew butter)
- Dried fruits (dates, apricots, raisins)

- Trail mix with nuts, seeds, and dried fruits
- Avocado toast with whole-grain bread
- Energy bars or protein bars

Cooking Instructions:
1. Portion out a serving of nuts, seeds, and dried fruits into small containers or snack bags for easy grab-and-go snacks.
2. Spread nut butter on whole-grain bread or toast and top with sliced avocado for a calorie-dense snack.
3. Choose energy bars or protein bars made with natural ingredients and minimal added sugars for a convenient snack option.

Cook Tips:
- Keep a stash of calorie-dense snacks on hand at home, at work, or when traveling to ensure you have access to nourishing snacks throughout the day.
- Pair your snacks with a source of protein or healthy fat to help keep you feeling full and satisfied between meals.

Nutritional Value:
- Calorie-dense snacks are an excellent choice for cancer patients looking to increase their calorie intake and support weight gain. Nuts and seeds are rich in healthy fats, protein, fiber, vitamins, and minerals, making them a nutrient-dense option for snacks. Nut butter provides additional healthy fats and protein, while dried fruits offer natural sweetness and quick energy. Enjoying calorie-dense snacks throughout the day can help cancer patients meet their nutritional needs and maintain or gain weight as needed.

Recipes for Maintaining a Healthy Weight

1. Balanced Main Meals

Ingredients:
- Lean protein (chicken breast, turkey breast, fish, tofu, tempeh)
- Whole grains (brown rice, quinoa, barley, farro)
- Vegetables (leafy greens, broccoli, cauliflower, bell peppers, zucchini)
- Healthy fats (avocado, olive oil, nuts, seeds)

Cooking Instructions:
1. Choose a lean protein source such as chicken breast, fish, tofu, or tempeh.
2. Pair the protein with a serving of whole grains like brown rice, quinoa, or barley.
3. Serve with a variety of colorful vegetables such as leafy greens, broccoli, cauliflower, bell peppers, or zucchini.
4. Add healthy fats to your meal by incorporating avocado slices, drizzling olive oil over vegetables, or sprinkling nuts or seeds on top.

Cook Tips:
- Aim to fill half of your plate with non-starchy vegetables, one-quarter with lean protein, and one-quarter with whole grains for a balanced and satisfying meal.
- Experiment with different cooking methods and flavor combinations to keep your meals interesting and enjoyable.

Nutritional Value:
- Balanced main meals provide cancer patients with a variety of nutrients essential

for overall health and well-being. Lean protein sources like chicken breast, fish, tofu, and tempeh provide amino acids necessary for tissue repair and muscle maintenance. Whole grains offer complex carbohydrates, fiber, vitamins, and minerals to support energy levels and digestive health. Vegetables are rich in vitamins, minerals, antioxidants, and fiber, which help support immune function and reduce inflammation. Healthy fats from avocado, olive oil, nuts, and seeds provide essential fatty acids and fat-soluble vitamins to support heart health and brain function. Enjoying balanced main meals can help cancer patients maintain a healthy weight and meet their nutritional needs for optimal health.

2. Low-Calorie Snacks

Ingredients:
- Fresh fruits (apples, oranges, berries, grapes, melon)
- Raw vegetables (carrot sticks, cucumber slices, cherry tomatoes, bell pepper strips)
- Air-popped popcorn
- Rice cakes or whole-grain crackers

- Greek yogurt or dairy-free yogurt alternative

Cooking Instructions:
1. Wash and prepare fresh fruits and vegetables by slicing or chopping them into bite-sized pieces.
2. Portion out a serving of air popped popcorn, rice cakes, or whole-grain crackers into small containers or snack bags for easy portion control.
3. Serve Greek yogurt or dairy-free yogurt alternative with fresh fruit or a drizzle of honey for a satisfying and nutritious snack option.

Cook Tips:
- Keep a variety of fresh fruits and vegetables on hand for quick and convenient snacking.
- Choose whole fruits and vegetables over fruit juices or processed snacks to maximize nutrient intake and minimize added sugars and preservatives.
- Pair low-calorie snacks with a source of protein or healthy fat to help keep you feeling full and satisfied between meals.

Nutritional Value:

- Low-calorie snacks are a smart choice for cancer patients looking to maintain a healthy weight and support overall health and well-being. Fresh fruits and vegetables are naturally low in calories and packed with essential vitamins, minerals, antioxidants, and fiber. Air-popped popcorn, rice cakes, and whole-grain crackers provide satisfying crunch and fiber to help keep you feeling full and satisfied. Greek yogurt or dairy-free yogurt alternative offers protein, probiotics, and calcium for bone health and digestive wellness. Enjoying low-calorie snacks throughout the day can help cancer patients manage their weight while still satisfying their hunger and nutritional needs.

These recipes for weight management offer delicious and nutritious options for cancer patients looking to maintain or achieve a healthy weight during treatment and recovery. Whether you're looking to gain weight or maintain your current weight, these recipes are designed to provide the nourishment and support you need to thrive. Incorporate these recipes into your meal plan to help support your weight management goals and enhance your overall health and well-being.

Recipes for Energy and Vitality

Maintaining energy levels and vitality is essential for cancer patients undergoing treatment and recovery. These recipes from "The Great Cancer Diet Cookbook" are specifically designed to provide high-energy snacks and meals that combat fatigue and promote overall well-being.

High-Energy Snacks and Meals

1. Nut Butter Energy Balls

Ingredients:
- 1 cup rolled oats
- 1/2 cup nut butter (almond butter, peanut butter, or cashew butter)
- 1/4 cup honey or maple syrup
- 1/4 cup ground flaxseeds or chia seeds
- 1/2 cup shredded coconut (unsweetened)
- 1/2 cup dark chocolate chips or cacao nibs
- 1 teaspoon vanilla extract
- Pinch of sea salt

Cooking Instructions:

1. In a large mixing bowl, combine rolled oats, nut butter, honey or maple syrup, ground flaxseeds or chia seeds, shredded coconut, dark chocolate chips or cacao nibs, vanilla extract, and a pinch of sea salt.

2. Mix well until all ingredients are evenly incorporated.

3. Using clean hands, roll the mixture into small balls, about 1 inch in diameter.

4. Place the energy balls on a baking sheet lined with parchment paper and chill in the refrigerator for at least 30 minutes to set.

5. Once chilled, store the nut butter energy balls in an airtight container in the refrigerator for up to two weeks.

Cook Tips:

- Customize your nut butter energy balls by adding other ingredients like dried fruits, nuts, seeds, or spices for extra flavor and nutrition.

- If the mixture is too dry, add a bit more nut butter or honey/maple syrup. If it's too wet, add more oats or shredded coconut to adjust the consistency.

Nutritional Value:
- Nut butter energy balls are a convenient and nutritious snack option for cancer patients needing an energy boost. Nut butter provides healthy fats and protein, while rolled oats offer complex carbohydrates and fiber for sustained energy. Ground flaxseeds or chia seeds contribute omega-3 fatty acids and additional fiber, while shredded coconut adds natural sweetness and texture. Dark chocolate chips or cacao nibs provide antioxidants and a touch of indulgence. Enjoying a couple of nut butter energy balls between meals can help maintain energy levels and provide essential nutrients for overall health and vitality.

2. Quinoa and Vegetable Stir-Fry

Ingredients:
- 1 cup quinoa, rinsed and drained
- 2 cups water or vegetable broth
- 1 tablespoon olive oil or coconut oil
- 2 cloves garlic, minced
- 1 onion, diced
- 2 carrots, sliced

- 1 bell pepper, sliced
- 1 zucchini, sliced
- 1 cup broccoli florets
- 1 cup snow peas or snap peas
- 1/4 cup soy sauce or tamari (gluten-free option)
- 1 tablespoon rice vinegar
- 1 tablespoon honey or maple syrup
- 1 teaspoon grated ginger
- Sesame seeds and chopped green onions for garnish (optional)

Cooking Instructions:
1. In a medium saucepan, combine quinoa and water or vegetable broth. Bring to a boil, then reduce heat to low, cover, and simmer for 15-20 minutes until quinoa is tender and water is absorbed. Remove from heat and let it sit, covered, for 5 minutes. Fluff with a fork and set aside.
2. In a large skillet or wok, heat olive oil or coconut oil over medium heat. Add minced garlic and diced onion, and sauté for 2-3 minutes until fragrant.
3. Add sliced carrots, bell pepper, zucchini, broccoli florets, and snow peas or snap peas to

the skillet. Cook for 5-7 minutes until vegetables are tender-crisp.

4. In a small bowl, whisk together soy sauce or tamari, rice vinegar, honey or maple syrup, and grated ginger to make the stir-fry sauce.

5. Pour the stir-fry sauce over the cooked vegetables in the skillet. Add cooked quinoa to the skillet and toss everything together until well combined and heated through.

6. Garnish with sesame seeds and chopped green onions if desired before serving.

Cook Tips:
- Feel free to customize your quinoa and vegetable stir-fry with your favorite vegetables and protein sources like tofu, tempeh, or cooked chicken or shrimp.
- Make a double batch of quinoa and store it in the refrigerator to use for quick and easy meals throughout the week.

Nutritional Value:
- Quinoa and vegetable stir-fry is a nutrient-rich and satisfying meal that provides a balance of carbohydrates, protein, and fiber to support energy levels and vitality.

Quinoa is a complete protein source and provides essential amino acids necessary for tissue repair and muscle maintenance. The colorful array of vegetables adds vitamins, minerals, antioxidants, and fiber to promote overall health and well-being. The stir-fry sauce adds flavor and depth to the dish while providing immune-boosting and anti-inflammatory benefits. Enjoying a serving of quinoa and vegetable stir-fry as a main meal can help cancer patients maintain energy levels and nourish their bodies with essential nutrients.

Foods to Combat Fatigue

1. Leafy Green Smoothies

Ingredients:
- 2 cups leafy greens (spinach, kale, Swiss chard)
- 1 ripe banana
- 1/2 cup frozen mixed berries (strawberries, blueberries, raspberries)
- 1 tablespoon almond butter or peanut butter

- 1 cup unsweetened almond milk or coconut water
- Optional add-ins: protein powder, chia seeds, flaxseeds, hemp seeds

Cooking Instructions:
1. In a blender, combine leafy greens, ripe banana, frozen mixed berries, almond butter or peanut butter, and unsweetened almond milk or coconut water.
2. Add any optional add-ins like protein powder, chia seeds, flaxseeds, or hemp seeds for extra nutrition.
3. Blend on high until smooth and creamy.
4. Taste and adjust sweetness or thickness by adding more banana or liquid if needed.
5. Pour the leafy green smoothie into glasses and serve immediately.

Cook Tips:
- Experiment with different combinations of leafy greens and fruits to find your favorite flavor profile.
- Add a handful of ice cubes to the blender for a chilled and refreshing smoothie.

Nutritional Value:
- Leafy green smoothies are a refreshing and nutrient-dense way to combat fatigue and boost energy levels. Leafy greens like spinach, kale, and Swiss chard are rich in vitamins, minerals, antioxidants, and phytonutrients that help support energy production and reduce inflammation. Mixed berries add natural sweetness and provide essential vitamins, minerals, and antioxidants to promote overall health and well-being. Almond butter or peanut butter adds healthy fats and protein to help keep you feeling full and satisfied. Enjoying a leafy green smoothie as a snack or meal can help cancer patients combat fatigue and nourish their bodies with essential nutrients.

2. Lentil and Quinoa Salad

Ingredients:
- 1 cup green or brown lentils, rinsed and drained
- 1/2 cup quinoa, rinsed and drained
- 2- 2 cups water or vegetable broth
- 1 tablespoon olive oil

- 2 cloves garlic, minced
- 1 onion, finely chopped
- 1 bell pepper, diced
- 1 cucumber, diced
- 1 cup cherry tomatoes, halved
- 1/4 cup fresh parsley, chopped
- 1/4 cup fresh cilantro, chopped
- Juice of 1 lemon
- 2 tablespoons apple cider vinegar
- Salt and pepper to taste

Cooking Instructions:

1. In a medium saucepan, combine lentils, quinoa, and water or vegetable broth. Bring to a boil, then reduce heat to low, cover, and simmer for 15-20 minutes until lentils and quinoa are tender and water is absorbed. Remove from heat and let it sit, covered, for 5 minutes. Fluff with a fork and set aside to cool.

2. In a large skillet, heat olive oil over medium heat. Add minced garlic and chopped onion, and sauté for 2-3 minutes until fragrant.

3. Add diced bell pepper to the skillet and cook for another 3-4 minutes until softened.

4. In a large mixing bowl, combine cooked lentils and quinoa with sautéed vegetables,

diced cucumber, halved cherry tomatoes, chopped parsley, and chopped cilantro.

5. Drizzle lemon juice and apple cider vinegar over the salad and toss everything together until well combined.

6. Season with salt and pepper to taste, and adjust seasoning if needed.

7. Chill the lentil and quinoa salad in the refrigerator for at least 30 minutes to allow flavors to meld before serving.

Cook Tips:

- To save time, you can use canned lentils and pre-cooked quinoa instead of cooking them from scratch. Just be sure to rinse canned lentils well before using.

- Customize your lentil and quinoa salad with your favorite vegetables, herbs, and dressings for variety and flavor.

Nutritional Value:

- Lentil and quinoa salad is a nutritious and energizing dish that provides a balance of protein, carbohydrates, fiber, vitamins, and minerals to combat fatigue and promote vitality. Lentils and quinoa are both excellent sources of plant-based protein and complex carbohydrates, which provide sustained energy and support muscle repair and recovery. The assortment of colorful vegetables adds vitamins, minerals, antioxidants, and fiber to support immune function and reduce inflammation. Fresh herbs like parsley and cilantro add flavor and phytonutrients, while lemon juice and apple cider vinegar provide a tangy kick and aid in digestion. Enjoying a serving of lentil and quinoa salad as a main meal or side dish can help cancer patients stay energized and nourished throughout the day.

These recipes for energy and vitality offer delicious and nutritious options for cancer patients looking to combat fatigue and boost overall well-being. Incorporate these recipes into your meal plan to help support your energy levels and vitality during treatment and recovery. Whether you're craving a high-energy snack or a nourishing meal, these recipes are sure to leave you feeling refreshed, revitalized, and ready to take on the day.

PART IV: EXPERT ADVICE AND RESOURCES

Expert Tips for Eating Well During Cancer Treatment

Eating well during cancer treatment is crucial for maintaining strength, managing side effects, and supporting overall health and well-being. Nutrition plays a significant role in the journey of cancer patients, and expert advice from nutritionists and oncologists can provide valuable guidance and support. In addition, personal stories and testimonials from cancer survivors offer insights and inspiration for navigating dietary challenges and embracing healing recipes. Here, we explore expert tips for eating well during cancer treatment, drawing on the expertise of professionals and the experiences of survivors.

Advice from Nutritionists and Oncologists

Nutritionists and oncologists play vital roles in helping cancer patients optimize their diets to support treatment outcomes and overall health. Here are some expert tips from these professionals:

1. **Focus on Nutrient-Dense Foods**: During cancer treatment, it's essential to prioritize nutrient-dense foods that provide essential vitamins, minerals, antioxidants, and protein. Aim to include a variety of colorful fruits and vegetables, whole grains, lean proteins, and healthy fats in your diet to ensure adequate nutrition.

2. **Stay Hydrated**: Maintaining hydration is crucial for managing side effects like nausea, vomiting, and dehydration during cancer treatment. Drink plenty of water throughout the day, and consider incorporating hydrating foods like soups, smoothies, and juicy fruits into your meal plan.

3. **Listen to Your Body:** Pay attention to your body's signals and adjust your diet based on how you're feeling. If you're experiencing appetite changes, nausea, or taste alterations, try small, frequent meals and bland, easy-to-digest foods. Experiment with

different flavors and textures to find what works best for you.

4. **Manage Side Effects**: Certain foods and dietary strategies can help manage common side effects of cancer treatment. For example, ginger may help alleviate nausea, while fiber-rich foods can help prevent constipation. Work with your healthcare team to develop a personalized nutrition plan tailored to your specific needs and treatment regimen.

5. **Supplement Wisely**: In some cases, cancer patients may require nutritional supplements to address deficiencies or support treatment-related side effects. Consult with your healthcare provider before taking any supplements, as they may interact with medications or affect treatment outcomes.

Personal Stories and Testimonials from Cancer Survivors

Personal stories and testimonials from cancer survivors offer unique perspectives and insights into the challenges and triumphs of navigating dietary changes during treatment. Here are some inspiring anecdotes and advice from individuals who have walked the path of cancer survivorship:

1. **Embrace Variety**: "During my cancer treatment, I found that embracing variety in my diet helped me stay motivated and nourished. Instead of focusing on what I couldn't eat, I focused on discovering new foods and flavors that supported my healing journey."

2. **Find Support**: "Navigating dietary changes during cancer treatment can be overwhelming, but finding support from loved ones, support groups, and online communities can make a world of difference. Don't be afraid to lean on others for guidance, encouragement, and recipe ideas."

3. **Listen to Your Cravings**: "Throughout my treatment, I learned to listen to my cravings and honor my body's needs. If I craved certain foods, I allowed myself to enjoy them in

moderation, knowing that nourishing my soul was just as important as nourishing my body."

4. **Practice Self-Care**: "Cancer treatment can take a toll on both the body and mind, so it's essential to prioritize self-care and nourishment during this time. Whether it's taking a warm bath, going for a gentle walk, or enjoying a nourishing meal, find ways to nourish yourself inside and out."

5. **Celebrate Small Victories**: "Recovering from cancer treatment is a journey filled with ups and downs, but it's important to celebrate every small victory along the way. Whether it's trying a new recipe, enjoying a meal with loved ones, or reaching a treatment milestone, take time to acknowledge and celebrate your progress."

Eating well during cancer treatment is a vital aspect of the healing journey, and expert advice from nutritionists and oncologists, combined with personal stories and testimonials from survivors, can provide valuable guidance and inspiration. By focusing on nutrient-dense foods, staying hydrated, listening to your body, managing side effects, and seeking support, cancer patients can optimize their diets to support treatment outcomes and overall well-being. Remember that every individual's journey is unique, so it's essential to find what works best for you and approach dietary changes with patience, compassion, and resilience. With the right support and mindset, embracing healing recipes and meal plans can be a transformative and empowering part of the cancer journey.

Resources and References

Navigating the complex landscape of cancer and nutrition can be challenging, but there are numerous resources available to support cancer patients and their caregivers. From recommended reading materials to informative websites and support organizations, these resources provide valuable information and guidance for incorporating healing recipes and meal plans into the cancer journey.

Recommended Reading on Nutrition and Cancer

1. *"Anticancer: A New Way of Life"* by David Servan-Schreiber: This groundbreaking book explores the relationship between diet, lifestyle, and cancer prevention, offering practical tips and insights for optimizing health and well-being.

2. *"The Cancer-Fighting Kitchen: Nourishing, Big-Flavor Recipes for Cancer Treatment and*

Recovery" by Rebecca Katz: Written by a chef and nutritionist, this cookbook offers flavorful recipes designed specifically for cancer patients undergoing treatment and recovery.

3. "*Radical Remission: Surviving Cancer Against All Odds*" by Kelly A. Turner, Ph.D.: Drawing on extensive research and interviews with cancer survivors, this book explores the factors that contribute to spontaneous remission and offers insights into holistic approaches to healing.

4. "*Cook for Your Life: Delicious, Nourishing Recipes for Before, During, and After Cancer Treatment*" by Ann Ogden Gaffney: This cookbook features easy-to-follow recipes tailored to the needs of cancer patients, with a focus on nutritious ingredients and flavorful dishes.

5. "*The Cancer Survivor's Guide: Foods That Help You Fight Back*" by Neal D. Barnard, MD, and Jennifer K. Reilly, RD: Written by a physician and registered dietitian, this comprehensive

guide provides evidence-based recommendations for diet and lifestyle changes to support cancer prevention and survivorship.

Useful Websites and Support Organizations

1. American Cancer Society (ACS): The ACS website offers a wealth of information on cancer prevention, treatment, and support services, including resources on nutrition and diet during cancer treatment.

2. National Cancer Institute (NCI): The NCI website provides evidence-based information on cancer research, treatment options, clinical trials, and supportive care resources, including guidance on nutrition and dietary recommendations for cancer patients.

3. CancerCare: CancerCare is a national nonprofit organization that provides free support services, including counseling, support groups, and educational resources for cancer patients, caregivers, and healthcare professionals.

4. The Cancer Nutrition Consortium (CNC): CNC is an organization dedicated to advancing the field of oncology nutrition through research, education, and advocacy. Their website offers resources on nutrition guidelines, patient education materials, and professional development opportunities for healthcare providers.

5. Cook for Your Life: Cook for Your Life is a nonprofit organization that provides free cooking classes, recipes, and nutrition resources specifically designed for cancer patients and survivors. Their website features a wide range of recipes, cooking tips, and meal planning tools to support individuals throughout their cancer journey.

Incorporating healing recipes and meal plans into the cancer journey can be a transformative and empowering experience. With the support of recommended reading materials, informative websites, and support organizations, cancer patients and their caregivers can access valuable resources and guidance to optimize nutrition, manage treatment-related side effects, and promote overall health and well-being. By embracing a holistic approach to cancer care that includes nourishing the body, mind, and spirit, individuals can navigate their cancer journey with resilience, strength, and hope.

Conclusion: Moving Forward with The Great Cancer Diet

As you reach the conclusion of The Great Cancer Diet Cookbook, you have embarked on a journey toward healing, nourishment, and empowerment. The recipes, meal plans, and expert advice within these pages have provided you with the tools and knowledge to support your body, mind, and spirit throughout the cancer journey. As you move forward, it's important to reflect on your progress, celebrate your successes, and continue your commitment to health and well-being.

Maintaining a Healthy Lifestyle Post-Treatment

As you transition from cancer treatment to survivorship, maintaining a healthy lifestyle is key to supporting your long-term health and vitality. Here are some tips for incorporating healthy habits into your post-treatment routine:

1. **Stay Active**: Regular physical activity is essential for maintaining strength, flexibility, and overall well-being. Aim for at least 30 minutes of moderate exercise most days of the week, and incorporate activities you enjoy, such as walking, swimming, or yoga.

2. **Follow a Balanced Diet**: Continue to prioritize nutrient-dense foods that support your body's healing and recovery. Focus on incorporating a variety of fruits, vegetables, whole grains, lean proteins, and healthy fats into your meals, and aim to limit processed foods, sugary snacks, and unhealthy fats.

3. **Stay Hydrated**: Drink plenty of water throughout the day to stay hydrated and support optimal health. Hydration is essential for digestion, circulation, and toxin removal, so aim to drink at least eight glasses of water daily, and adjust your intake based on your activity level and climate.

4. **Get Plenty of Sleep**: Adequate sleep is essential for healing, immune function, and

overall health. Aim for 7-9 hours of quality sleep each night, and establish a relaxing bedtime routine to promote restful sleep, such as reading, gentle stretching, or listening to calming music.

5. **Manage Stress**: Find healthy ways to manage stress and cultivate a sense of peace and relaxation in your daily life. Practice mindfulness meditation, deep breathing exercises, or gentle yoga to reduce stress and promote emotional well-being.

Continuing Your Nutritional Journey

Your journey toward optimal health and well-being is ongoing, and there is always more to learn and explore. Here are some ways to continue your nutritional journey and deepen your understanding of the connection between diet and cancer:

1. **Explore New Recipes**: Continue to experiment with new recipes and ingredients that support your health and well-being. Try incorporating more plant-based foods,

antioxidant-rich spices, and healing herbs into your meals to boost flavor and nutritional value.

2. **Stay Informed:** Stay up-to-date on the latest research and recommendations related to cancer prevention, treatment, and survivorship. Follow reputable sources such as the American Cancer Society, National Cancer Institute, and Cancer Nutrition Consortium for evidence-based information and resources.

3. **Share Your Knowledge**: Share your knowledge and experience with others who may benefit from your insights. Whether it's through supporting friends and family members facing cancer, participating in community events, or advocating for policy changes to support cancer prevention and treatment, your voice can make a difference.

4. **Seek Support**: Continue to seek support from healthcare professionals, support groups, and online communities to help you navigate the challenges and triumphs of the

cancer journey. Connect with others who understand what you're going through and share your experiences, challenges, and victories along the way.

 Final Thoughts and Encouragement

As you close the pages of The Great Cancer Diet Cookbook, remember that you are not alone on your journey. You have a wealth of resources, support, and knowledge at your disposal to help you navigate the ups and downs of cancer treatment and survivorship. Embrace the power of healing foods, nourishing recipes, and supportive communities to empower yourself on your path to health and well-being.

In the words of cancer survivor and advocate, Lance Armstrong, "Pain is temporary. Quitting lasts forever." Let this mantra guide you as you face the challenges of cancer with courage, resilience, and determination. With each nourishing meal, each step toward wellness, and each moment of connection with others, you are affirming your commitment to health, vitality, and life.

As you move forward on your journey, know that you have the strength, wisdom, and support to overcome any obstacle that comes your way. Trust in your body's ability to heal and thrive, and never lose sight of the hope and possibility that lie ahead. You are a survivor, a warrior, and an inspiration to all who know you. Keep shining your light, sharing your story, and embracing the power of healing one meal at a time.

In conclusion, The Great Cancer Diet Cookbook is more than just a collection of recipes; it is a guidebook for healing, nourishment, and empowerment. Through its pages, you have discovered the transformative power of food to support your body's healing and recovery. From nutrient-dense smoothies to comforting soups to indulgent desserts, these recipes offer a wealth of delicious options to nourish your body, mind, and spirit throughout the cancer journey.

As you embark on your own culinary adventure, remember the importance of balance, variety, and moderation in your diet. Listen to your body's cues, honor your cravings, and prioritize self-care and well-being in all that you do. With the guidance of nutritionists, oncologists, and fellow survivors, you have the knowledge and support you need to make informed choices and embrace a healthy lifestyle post-treatment.

As you continue your nutritional journey, know that you are not alone. You are part of a vibrant community of individuals who are navigating similar challenges and triumphs. Lean on each other for support, share your experiences and insights, and celebrate every step forward on your path to health and wellness.

In closing, remember that healing is not a destination; it is a journey. Embrace the process, stay true to yourself, and trust in the power of food to nourish, heal, and transform.

With The Great Cancer Diet Cookbook as your guide, may you find strength, inspiration, and hope in every meal, and may your journey be filled with health, happiness, and abundance.

APPENDIX

Appendix A: Nutritional Information

In The Great Cancer Diet Cookbook, we understand the importance of providing detailed nutritional information for each recipe to help cancer patients make informed dietary choices. This appendix offers a comprehensive breakdown of the nutritional content of our healing recipes, along with guidance on understanding nutritional labels to support your health and well-being.

Detailed Nutritional Breakdown of Each Recipe

Each recipe in The Great Cancer Diet Cookbook is carefully crafted to provide nourishment, flavor, and healing benefits for cancer patients. Here's a breakdown of the key nutritional components you'll find in our recipes:

1. **Macronutrients:** Our recipes include information on the amounts of protein, carbohydrates, and fats per serving. Protein is essential for building and repairing tissues, while carbohydrates provide energy and fiber. Healthy fats,

such as omega-3 fatty acids, support brain health and reduce inflammation.

2. **Micronutrients:** We also provide details on the vitamins and minerals present in each recipe. These micronutrients play crucial roles in supporting immune function, promoting healthy cell growth, and protecting against oxidative stress. Common micronutrients found in our recipes include vitamin C, vitamin A, iron, calcium, and potassium.

3. **Caloric Content:** Understanding the caloric content of each recipe can help cancer patients manage their energy intake and maintain a healthy weight during treatment. Our recipes offer balanced calorie counts to support overall health and well-being.

4. **Fiber Content:** Fiber is important for digestive health and can help alleviate constipation, a common side effect of cancer treatment. Our recipes include information on fiber content to help patients meet their daily fiber needs.

5. **Antioxidants and Phytochemicals:** Many of our recipes are rich in antioxidants and phytochemicals, which have been shown to have anti-inflammatory and cancer-fighting properties. Ingredients such as colorful fruits and vegetables, herbs, spices, and whole grains provide a wealth of these beneficial compounds.

Understanding Nutritional Labels

In addition to the nutritional information provided for each recipe, it's important for cancer patients to understand how to interpret nutritional labels on packaged foods. Here are some key points to keep in mind:

1. **Serving Size:** Pay attention to the serving size listed on the label, as all of the nutritional information is based on this serving size. Be mindful of portion sizes to avoid overeating and to ensure accurate nutrient intake.
2. **Total Calories:** The total number of calories per serving is listed on the label. This information can help you track

your daily calorie intake and make informed decisions about portion sizes.

3. **Macronutrients:** Look for information on protein, carbohydrates, and fats per serving. Aim for a balanced mix of these macronutrients in your diet to support your nutritional needs.

4. **Ingredients List:** Scan the ingredients list to identify any potential allergens or additives. Choose foods with simple, whole food ingredients and avoid products with added sugars, artificial preservatives, and unhealthy fats.

5. **% Daily Value (%DV):** The %DV indicates how much of a nutrient one serving of the food provides relative to the recommended daily intake. Aim for foods that provide higher %DV for essential nutrients like vitamins, minerals, and fiber.

6. **Nutrient Claims:** Pay attention to nutrient claims such as "low-fat," "sugar-free," or "high-fiber." While these claims can be helpful, it's important to read the full nutritional

label to ensure that the product aligns with your dietary goals and needs.

By providing detailed nutritional information for each recipe and guidance on understanding nutritional labels, The Great Cancer Diet Cookbook empowers cancer patients to make informed dietary choices to support their health and well-being. Whether you're looking to increase your intake of nutrient-rich foods, manage side effects of treatment, or maintain a healthy weight, our recipes and nutritional guidance are designed to help you on your journey to healing.

As you incorporate these healing recipes and meal plans into your diet, remember to listen to your body, honor your cravings, and prioritize self-care and nourishment. By nourishing your body with wholesome, nourishing foods and staying informed about your nutritional needs, you can support your body's natural healing processes and optimize your overall health and well-being during and after cancer treatment

Appendix B: Meal Plan Templates

Meal planning is an essential aspect of maintaining a healthy diet, especially for cancer patients who may face unique dietary challenges. In this appendix, we provide sample meal plans for different dietary needs, along with customizable weekly meal planning templates to help you create nourishing and balanced meals tailored to your preferences and nutritional requirements.

Sample Meal Plans for Different Dietary Needs

1. General Cancer-Fighting Meal Plan:

- Breakfast: Green Power Smoothie

- Snack: Almond and Date Energy Balls

- Lunch: Kale and Quinoa Salad with Lemon Dressing

- Snack: Veggie Chips with Avocado and White Bean Dip

- Dinner: Baked Salmon with Asparagus

- Dessert: Dark Chocolate Avocado Mousse

2. **Plant-Based Meal Plan:**

- Breakfast: Berry Antioxidant Smoothie

- Snack: Hummus and Veggie Sticks

- Lunch: Chickpea and Spinach Curry

- Snack: Roasted Chickpeas

- Dinner: Quinoa-Stuffed Bell Peppers

- Dessert: Berry Parfait

3. **Gluten-Free Meal Plan:**

- Breakfast: Quinoa and Berry Breakfast Bowl

- Snack: Rice Cakes with Almond Butter

- Lunch: Spinach and Avocado Salad

- Snack: Mixed Nuts

- Dinner: Black Bean and Sweet Potato Enchiladas

- Dessert: Baked Apples with Cinnamon

4. Dairy-Free Meal Plan:

- Breakfast: Oatmeal with Nuts and Seeds

- Snack: Coconut Yogurt with Berries

- Lunch: Lentil and Vegetable Soup

- Snack: Fresh Fruit Salad

- Dinner: Grilled Veggie Wrap with Hummus

- Dessert: Grilled Pineapple with Honey

Appendix C: Ingredient Substitutions

Ingredient substitutions are a handy tool for adapting recipes to fit specific dietary needs or preferences. In this appendix, we provide a list of common substitutes for allergy-friendly cooking, along with creative alternatives for key ingredients to help you create delicious and nutritious meals that cater to your individual needs.

Common Substitutes for Allergy-Friendly Cooking

1. Dairy Substitutes:

   - Coconut milk or almond milk can be used in place of cow's milk in recipes.

   - Vegan butter or coconut oil can replace butter in baking recipes.

- Nutritional yeast can add a cheesy flavor to dishes without the need for dairy cheese.

2. Gluten Substitutes:

- Gluten-free flour blends made from rice flour, almond flour, or coconut flour can replace wheat flour in baking recipes.

- Quinoa, rice, or corn pasta can be used instead of traditional wheat pasta.

- Gluten-free oats can be used in place of regular oats in oatmeal and baked goods.

3. Egg Substitutes:

- Flaxseed or chia seed gel can be used as a binding agent in place of eggs in baking recipes.

- Mashed banana or applesauce can add moisture and structure to baked goods without the need for eggs.

- Silken tofu can be blended and used as a creamy substitute for eggs in recipes like quiches and custards.

Creative Alternatives for Key Ingredients

1. Sweeteners:

- Maple syrup, honey, or agave nectar can be used as alternatives to refined sugar in recipes.

- Medjool dates or date paste can add natural sweetness to desserts and baked goods.

2. **Fats:**

- Avocado, mashed banana, or Greek yogurt can be used as substitutes for butter or oil in baking recipes.

- Nut butters, such as almond or cashew butter, can add richness and flavor to dishes without the need for added fats.

3. **Flavor Enhancers:**

- Tamari or coconut aminos can be used as gluten-free alternatives to soy sauce in recipes.

- Herbs, spices, and citrus zest can add depth and complexity to dishes without the need for excess salt or sugar.

In conclusion, the appendices of The Great Cancer Diet Cookbook provide valuable resources and tools to support cancer patients in their dietary journey. From sample meal plans and customizable templates to ingredient substitutions and comprehensive indexes, these appendices offer practical guidance and inspiration for creating nourishing and delicious meals that promote healing and well-being.

www.ingramcontent.com/pod-product-compliance
Lightning Source LLC
Chambersburg PA
CBHW070822250726